# Tai Chi Chuan Common Knowledge

The Definitive Textbook of Tai Chi Fundamentals

Li Peiyun, Kevin Else

Library of Congress Control Number: 2025900078

ISBN: 979-8-9923011-2-0 (Hardcover)

ISBN: 979-8-9923011-0-6 (Paperback)

ISBN: 979-8-9923011-1-3 (eBook)

Publisher: Standing Pole LLC, Media, PA 19063

Copyright © 2025 by Li Peiyun and Kevin Else

First edition 2025

All rights reserved.

No part of this publication may be reproduced, distributed, or transmitted in any form or by any means, including but not limited to photocopying, recording, or other electronic or mechanical methods, without the prior written permission of the publisher, except in the case of brief quotations embodied in critical articles and reviews. The information provided in this book is for educational purposes only. The exercises and strategies discussed are not a substitute for professional medical advice. Prior to beginning any new exercise regimen, including Tai Chi, consult with a healthcare professional to ensure it is appropriate for your specific health conditions and abilities. The author and publisher disclaim any liability for injury or damage that may result from following the instructions contained in this book. Always practice safely and within the limits of your own abilities.

Book Cover Design by Kevin Else

Cover Photography by Eugene Colucci

Illustrations by an unknown Chinese illustrator as modified by Kevin Else

Original Publication Credit: The original textbook was compiled by Zhou Renfeng and published by the People's Sports Publishing House in June 1978 (Printed by Tianjin First Printing Factory, distributed by Xinhua Bookstore Beijing Branch).

# Contents

| | |
|---|---|
| Acknowledgements | X |
| Translator's Note | XI |
| Preface | XIII |
| 1. Knowledge and Key Points of Tai Chi Chuan | 1 |

    1. Who created Tai Chi Chuan?

    2. How many types of Tai Chi Chuan are there?

    3. Why is it called Tai Chi Chuan?

    4. How Many Types of Hand Forms Are There in Tai Chi Chuan?

    5. What are the requirements for the shoulders, elbows, and wrists in Tai Chi Chuan?

    6. What Are the Requirements for the Head and Neck in Tai Chi Chuan?

    7. What requirements does Tai Chi have on the mouth?

    8. What are the requirements for the chest and back in Tai Chi Chuan?

    9. Is it about "relaxed abdomen" or "engaged abdomen"? Can practicing Tai Chi Chuan lead to a big belly?

    10. Why does Tai Chi Chuan particularly emphasize the waist?

11. What are the Tai Chi Chuan Requirements for the Buttocks and Groin Area?

12. What are the requirements for Legs in Tai Chi Chuan?

13. What are the Types of Stances in Tai Chi Chuan?

14. What is the Essence of Tai Chi Chuan Footwork.

15. What are the leg techniques of Tai Chi? How to make independent legs stand stable?

16. What is The Practice and Significance of Stance Training in Tai Chi Chuan?

17. What are the main techniques of Tai Chi?

18. How to pay attention to your eyes when practicing Tai Chi Chuan?

19. What are the Body Methods in Tai Chi Chuan.

20. Why does Tai Chi Chuan practice place special emphasis on relaxation?

21. How to understand the relationship between movement and stillness in Tai Chi?

22. What is The Relationship and Synergistic Effect of Relaxation and Stillness?

23. What does "Qi" refer to, and does it offer any benefits?

24. What are the Benefits of Mind-led Movement in Tai Chi Chuan?

25. How can we achieve "Unity of Mind and Qi"?

26. How to Achieve "Rooted in the Feet, Generated in the Legs, Governed by the Waist, Manifested in the Fingers.

27. How many breathing methods are there in Tai Chi?

28. Is the statement "breathing in and out of the mouth" correct?

29. Is the statement "movements and breathing must be integrated" correct?

30. How should breathing coordinate with movements in Tai Chi Chuan?

31. How do you Understand 'Opening with Inhalation, Closing with Exhalation' versus 'Closing with Inhalation, Opening with Exhalation'

32. What Are the Benefits of Natural Deep Breathing in Tai Chi Chuan?

33. What is "Qi sinking in Dantian" and How Is It Practiced and Understood?

34. How Does Tai Chi Chuan Benefit the Skin?

35. How to Understand 'Everywhere There Is Emptiness and Fullness'?

36. What is Double-Weighting? How Can It Be Avoided?

37. How to Understand and Achieve 'Coordination Between Upper and Lower Body, Whole-Body Harmony'?

38. How to understand and achieve "internal and external harmony"?

39. How do we understand the phrase: "Where there is up, there is down; where there is front, there is back; where there is left, there is right"?

40. How to Understand and Achieve 'Continuity without Interruption'?

41. How to Master the pace in Tai Chi?

42. What is meant by "light, agile, sinking, and stable" and "hardness and softness complementing each other"?

43. What is the Significance of Circular and Spiral Movements in Tai Chi Chuan.

44. Why is Tai Chi Chuan Also Known as the Thirteen Postures?

2. Physiological Hygiene in Tai Chi Chuan Practice                100

1. What kind of environment is suitable for practicing Tai Chi Chuan?

2. When are the Optimal Times for Daily Tai Chi Practice?

3. How should one Gauge the Correct Exercise Intensity in Tai Chi Chuan Practice?

4. What should be the Guidelines for Practicing Tai Chi Chuan for Individuals with Weakness or Chronic Illness?

5. What preparations should be made before practicing Tai Chi?

6. What should one Do After Completing a Tai Chi Chuan Session?

7. What to do if your legs feel sore when learning Tai Chi Chuan?

8. Can one Practice Tai Chi Chuan During Menstruation, Pregnancy, and Lactation?

9. How Should One Manage Their Diet When Practicing Tai Chi Chuan?

10. Is It Correct to Avoid Urination or Defecation Before Morning Tai Chi Practice?

11. Why Do Some People's Hands Get Cold After Practicing Tai Chi in Winter?"

12. What Causes Shaking During Tai Chi Practice and How to Prevent It?

13. Is it good to make sounds while practicing Tai chi Chuan? What is the impact of talking while practicing?

14. How Should We View the Concept of "Promoting Longevity and Eternal Youth" in Tai Chi Chuan?

15. Is it possible to practice other physical activities while learning Tai Chi Chuan?

16. Why do people with neurasthenia benefit significantly from practicing Tai Chi Chuan, and what should they be mindful of?

17. What should patients with pulmonary tuberculosis be aware of when practicing Tai Chi Chuan?

18. Can people with bronchitis practice Tai Chi Chuan, and what should they be mindful of?

19. How can one prevent catching a cold while practicing Tai Chi Chuan?

20. Why is Tai Chi Chuan effective in preventing and treating heart disease, and what should heart patients be mindful of when practicing?

21. What should individuals with hypertension pay attention to when practicing Tai Chi Chuan?

22. Why is Tai Chi Chuan effective in preventing and treating flat feet?

23. What should arthritis patients consider when practicing Tai Chi Chuan?

24. Is there any benefit for manual laborers in practicing Tai Chi Chuan?

25. What are the benefits of practicing Tai Chi Chuan from a young age?

3. Tai Chi Chuan Push Hands, Implements, and Instruction   137

1. What is Push Hands and Sensing Energy?

2. What Does "Jin" Refer to in Tai Chi Chuan? How to Enhance "Internal Jin"?

3. What are Sticking, Adhering, Connecting, and Following? What Common Issues Arise in Push Hands?

4. What is the Dialectical Relationship Between Curved and Straight Forces in Tai Chi Chuan Push Hands?

5. Why is it said that "to retreat is to prepare to advance" in Push Hands?

6. What does "Gold Shoulders, Silver Chest, Tin Wax Belly" mean in Push Hands?

7. Why is the Upward Pressing Force More Effective in Pushing the Opponent?

8. How can you stand firm when pushing hands?

9. What does "Lightness Above, Solidity Below, Agility in the Middle" mean?

10. What Weapons are Included in the Tai Chi System?

11. What Challenges are Encountered in Learning Tai Chi Chuan?

12. What teaching methods are commonly used in Tai Chi Chuan?

13. How to use Explanation and Demonstration in teaching Tai Chi Chuan?

14. What Does It Mean to Practice or Frame the Framework? Is the Method of "Seeking Extension First, Then Compactness" Correct?

4. Selection and Practice of Tai Chi Chuan     163

   1. Preparatory Stance

   2. Rising and Falling (Cupping and Pressing)

   3. Opening and Closing

   4. Vertical Circular Elements

   5. Horizontal Circular Elements in Tai Chi Chuan

   6. Diagonal Circular Elements (Parting the Wild Horse's Mane)

   7. Brush Knee-Circling Step

   8. Cloudy Hands

   9. Kicking

   10. One Leg Standing

   11. Horse Stance with Palm Push

   12. Closing Form

About the Translators     182

# Acknowledgements

I am deeply grateful to Master Don Hawkins, an 8th Degree Black Belt in Isshin-Ryu Karate-do and esteemed inductee into the Isshin-Ryu Hall of Fame, for his invaluable assistance in reviewing this book and offering insightful suggestions. His expertise and guidance have significantly enhanced the quality and accuracy of this work.

I would also like to express my heartfelt appreciation to my family for their unwavering support and patience throughout the writing process. Their encouragement has been a constant source of motivation.

Finally, I am indebted to my readers and fellow students, whose interest and enthusiasm for this subject continue to inspire me. It is my hope that this book will contribute meaningfully to their understanding and appreciation of the amazing art of Tai Chi Chuan.

Kevin Else

January 2025

# Translator's Note

The translation of this book marks a significant advancement in the English-language understanding of Tai Chi Chuan (also referred to as Tai Chi or Tai Ji). Originally conceived as a companion piece to the previously published Tai Chi manual, "Tai Chi Common Sense: Questions and Answers" by Zhang Wenyuan, this book, first published in China in 1978, carries forward the tradition of imparting invaluable knowledge. My introduction to this manual came through my esteemed sifu and coach, Master Li Peiyun, with whom I've had the privilege of training with since 1999. Master Li's profound insights into the art have enriched my understanding in ways unmatched by any written text. It was our mutual belief that translating this work into English would be a valuable contribution to the English-speaking martial arts community. The three (3) year long process of compiling the information imparted in this book is fully described in Zhou Renfeng's original Preface.

In translating this text, I have chosen NOT to include some sections which contain political language and/or references to political leaders, despite their historical relevance, these statements add little to the understanding of Tai Chi. My decision stems from a desire to provide readers with an understanding of Tai Chi without the political baggage of the 1960s and 1970s. However, I understand that these redactions may not be acceptable to all readers, and I apologize if it detracts from your experience with this translation.

You will notice the numbering of Illustrations restarts in Chapter 4. I chose to keep the numbering system used in the original text as it helped reduce the number of errors in the overall text. In addition, in keeping with Chinese naming conventions, this English translation maintains the traditional order of personal names, with surnames appearing first.

I recognize the importance of transparency in the translation process, and I hope that this brief explanation sheds light on the considerations and choices made during the translation of this work.

This translation attempts to not only convey the original content but also (I hope) encapsulate the essence of Tai Chi Chuan's approach to health and well-being, presented in a manner that I trust will resonate with both beginning and advanced practitioners and those with a scholarly interest in this ancient martial art and teaching technique. I have found the text to be invaluable in helping to correct some of my misunderstandings and inadequacies in the art of Tai Chi Chuan. We believe this textbook will provide similar benefits to the reader, both beginners and advanced practitioners alike.

As with any translation, the responsibility for accuracy lies with the translator. Master Li's explanations and corrections have been invaluable and his profound knowledge and understanding far exceed the limits of this textbook. The responsibility for any inaccuracies are mine and any helpful suggestions or corrections from the reader are welcome.

Kevin Else

January 2025

# Preface

To assist the vast majority of the populace in better engaging in Tai Chi Chuan practice and addressing the issues encountered during practice, this book was compiled. Prior to its writing, the People's Sports Publishing House commissioned Wu Yaowen, Zhou Yuanlong, and the editors to seek opinions from workers, peasants, and soldiers in Taiyuan, Shanghai, Xi'an, and other places. Based on these opinions and a review of both ancient and modern Tai Chi Chuan materials, the editors absorbed the main content of "Common Questions and Answers in Tai Chi Chuan" (authored by Zhang Wenyuan) previously published by the People's Sports Publishing House to write the first draft.

After the first draft was completed, feedback was sought from students in teaching sessions, leading to the first revision. Subsequently, comrades such as Wu Yaowen and Zhou Yuanlong reviewed the manuscript, and a second revision was made based on their suggestions. After the second revision, to further solicit opinions and meet teaching needs, Xi'an Institute of Physical Education printed twenty thousand copies, which, following further feedback from a broad spectrum of workers, peasants, and soldiers, led to a third revision. The Xi'an Institute of Physical Education, Shanxi Machine Tool Factory, Shanghai Municipal Sports Committee, Shanghai Sports Palace, Hebei Normal University, Shaanxi Provincial Sports Committee, and Qingdao Municipal Sanitation and Epidemic Prevention Station provided significant support in soliciting opinions and during the compilation process. We also thank comrades Zhou Yuanlong and Wu Yaowen for their assistance in reviewing and revising the manuscript.

Over the past three years, despite several rounds of soliciting feedback and making revisions during the writing process, shortcomings and errors are difficult to avoid due to the limitations of the editors' expertise. We welcome corrections from our readers.

Xi'an Institute of Physical Education, Zhou Renfeng

February 1977

# Chapter One

## Knowledge and Key Points of Tai Chi Chuan

### 1. Who created Tai Chi Chuan?

Whether it's the Tai Chi Chuan passed down from Chen Village in Wenxian County, Henan, or the "Tongbei Boxing" passed down from Hongdong, Shanxi (preliminary investigation suggests it might be the lost "Long Fist" from Chen Village in Wenxian County, Henan), they are all related to the 32 forms of boxing summarized by Qi Jiguang (1528-1587) of the Ming Dynasty. Many of the form names are the same, and Tai Chi Chuan adopted 29 of the 32 forms, showing a very obvious inheritance relationship. Qi Jiguang himself admitted that his boxing manual was compiled based on sixteen folk martial arts styles. History cannot be reversed. The origin of Tai Chi Chuan, this national cultural heritage, can only be the creation of generations of Chinese people, continuously enriched and developed through social practice.

### 2. How many types of Tai Chi Chuan are there?

The varieties of Tai Chi Chuan are numerous. Looking at the currently popular types alone, they can generally be divided into three systems based on the size of the form, or into five categories based on the characteristics and styles of the movements.

## Three Systems:

1. **Large Frame:** Represented by Chen Style Tai Chi Chuan, Yang Style Tai Chi Chuan, the Eighty-Eight Forms Tai Chi Chuan, and Simplified Tai Chi Chuan, which often utilize a large frame. The characteristic of the large frame is that the movements are expansive and graceful, combining agility and stability.

2. **Medium Frame:** Represented by Wu (Hao) Style Tai Chi Chuan, which has a moderately sized frame and specializes in softening techniques.

3. **Small Frame:** Represented by Sun Style and Wu Style Tai Chi Chuan, characterized by compact and precise movements, with lively steps and agile body movements.

## Five Categories:

1. **Yang Style Tai Chi Chuan:** Smooth and gentle, expansive and graceful.

2. **Chen Style Tai Chi Chuan:** Integrates hardness with softness, and fast with slow movements. It includes new frame, old frame, large frame, and small frame variations.

3. **Wu (Hao) Style Tai Chi Chuan:** Soft and compact, with a moderate size.

4. **Wu Style Tai Chi Chuan:** Features flexible movements and light footwork.

5. **Sun Style Tai Chi Chuan:** Similar to Wu Style in characteristics, it emphasizes opening and closing movements, compactness, and

lively steps with an agile body.

The categories listed above are a preliminary classification. If we were to detail further, there are several other styles, each with its unique features. The Simplified Tai Chi Chuan and the Eighty-Eight Forms Tai Chi Chuan have been mainly adapted by the National Sports Commission from the most widely practiced Yang Style Tai Chi Chuan. Practitioners can choose based on their physical condition, age, and preferences, and can also adjust their practice flexibly according to circumstances. For example, a small frame can be adapted into a medium or large frame, and likewise, a large frame can be adapted into a medium or small frame. Elderly individuals or those with physical weaknesses or illnesses who practice Chen Style Tai Chi Chuan can also omit the more overt forceful and stomping actions.

# 3. Why is it called Tai Chi Chuan?

The naming of Tai Chi Chuan is subject to various interpretations. The following explanations are offered for consideration:

### The Tai Chi Diagram and the Duality of Movement:

The Tai Chi diagram represents the duality of Yin and Yang, and Tai Chi Chuan distinguishes between the substantial and the insubstantial in every movement. This is why it is called Tai Chi Chuan. It implies that practicing Tai Chi Chuan without distinguishing between the substantial and the insubstantial does not meet the requirements implied by the name itself.

### The Tai Chi Diagram and the Principle of Relaxation:

The Tai Chi diagram divides Yin and Yang, and Tai Chi Chuan emphasizes total body relaxation, with the head as if suspended from above, chest slightly concave and back slightly convex, shoulders sunk and elbows drooping, and energy concentrated in the dantian. This achieves a state of being 'empty' above and 'solid' below (especially with an 'empty' chest and 'solid' abdomen), hence the name Tai Chi Chuan. Thus, if one cannot achieve this state of 'empty' above and 'solid' below, the lower stance will not be stable, which also contradicts the meaning of the name.

## The Circular Nature of Tai Chi:

The Tai Chi diagram is circular, and the movements of Tai Chi Chuan are mostly arc-shaped or circular, hence the name. It is important in practice to carefully observe whether the movements are circular and arc-shaped. Initially, movements may appear more angular, establishing a framework that gradually becomes more rounded. This approach has been proven feasible through practice by many.

## The Concept of "Tai Chi" in Ancient Times:

In ancient times, the initial separation of heaven and earth was referred to as "Tai Chi," also known as "The Beginning." Tai Chi Chuan was thus named to imply it as the "earliest" or "supreme" form of boxing, indicating a high regard for this martial art. Tai Chi Chuan is esteemed for its health benefits, disease prevention and treatment capabilities, and is suitable for men and women of all ages. Its movements are graceful and gentle, allowing for continuous deepening of skill without losing interest. Therefore, valuing, studying, and promoting Tai Chi Chuan as a precious cultural heritage is appropriate and advocated. However, from a historical materialism perspective, it is not the "earliest" or "supreme," as it needs to evolve and improve. Furthermore, other forms of martial arts also have their merits and characteristics compared to Tai Chi Chuan. Hence, such a proposition may seem sectarian and is inappropriate.

# 4. How Many Types of Hand Forms Are There in Tai Chi Chuan?

In Tai Chi Chuan, hand forms are categorized into three (3) types: palm, fist, and hook, with palm techniques being the primary focus within the routines.

## Palm

The term "palm" has both broad and narrow meanings: in the broad sense, it refers to the entire hand as long as the fingers are extended; in the narrow sense, it refers to the part of the hand from the wrist joint to beyond the base joint of the little finger, where the outer edge of the hand has more muscle. Tai Chi Chuan encompasses both meanings for the palm.

Different styles of Tai Chi Chuan have slightly different requirements for the palm. For example, in Yang, Wu (Hao), and Sun styles, the palm should be naturally extended without forcefully spreading or clenching the fingers, allowing a tiny gap between them. When one's skill is profound, the distinction between the substantial and insubstantial should also be reflected in the palm. For instance, when extending the hand forward, before the extension, the palm should be slightly cupped, storing energy without expanding, representing the insubstantial palm. During the extension, gradually reduce the cupping, transitioning from insubstantial to substantial; at the endpoint, the cupping becomes shallow or nearly disappears, with slightly spread fingers and a settled wrist (dropped wrist), and the root of the palm protruding slightly forward to aid the extending momentum, focusing the intent and energy on the fingertips, known as the substantial palm. When retracting the palm, it transitions from extended to reserved, returning to a slightly cupped position, known as moving from substantial to insubstantial. In Wu (Hao) Style Tai Chi Chuan, the substantial palm nearly eliminates the cupping or protrudes forward; in Chen Style, the palm appears slightly protruded from the fingers to the wrist (vertically) and concave from the thumb to the little finger (horizontally).

The movement of the palm is part of the whole body movement; thus, the transitions between substantial and insubstantial in the palm should match the overall movement. The hand should coordinate with the complete movements of the waist, legs, and feet.

### Fist

The fist is formed by curling the four fingers close together, with the thumb resting horizontally on the second phalanges of the index and middle fingers. If the purpose is for healing, the fist should generally be held loosely; if practicing a more forceful form of Tai Chi Chuan, the grip should alternate between tight and loose, clenching tightly at the moment of force application and then quickly relaxing to a loose state. When extending the fist, it should align straight with the forearm without twisting outward or inward, as twisting can cause wrist tension and impede the flow of Qi and blood.

### Hook

There are two (2) types of hooks: one where the tips of the thumb, index, and little fingers meet, with the middle and ring fingers closing in towards them; the other involves all five fingertips coming together. Either method is acceptable, but it's important to keep the fingers naturally close, the wrist relaxed, and the whole hand naturally drooping.

It must be noted that these three hand forms in Tai Chi Chuan often change throughout the practice. During transitions, movements should be slow and not too rapid or forceful (except when applying forceful energy), especially ensuring the wrist remains relaxed.

## 5. What are the requirements for the shoulders, elbows, and wrists in Tai Chi Chuan?

In the upper limb posture of Tai Chi Chuan, the most important aspects are "dropping the shoulders and elbows" and "settling the wrists," with the key emphasis on relaxing or dropping the shoulders. The shoulder is an extremely crucial part of the upper body, connecting the upper arm with the scapula and collarbone through the deltoid muscle, linking the thoracic and lumbar spine to the humerus with the latissimus dorsi, and joining the humerus, sternum, and collarbone with the pectoralis major.

Therefore, to facilitate full arm movement, which simultaneously involves chest and back movements, the shoulders must be highly relaxed. Only then can the upper body, chest, and back fully relax, achieving a state where the upper body is light and agile, and the lower body is solid and stable. Shoulders should be relaxed and flexible, and the elbow joints must maintain a slight bend, implying a drooping intention. This facilitates better relaxation of the shoulder joints, sinking the energy into the lower abdomen, and easing bending, extending, and transitioning between substantial and insubstantial. While the elbows droop, they should also slightly open outward, allowing for better relaxation of the pectoralis major and maintaining some space under the armpits, enhancing shoulder joint flexibility. However, the elbows should not flare out noticeably, avoiding the appearance of "showing the elbow" (also called "raising the elbow"). This is what people refer to when they say "sometimes the elbow is not seen in front of the chest." "Being seen" means "showing the elbow." If the shoulders and elbows are not dropped, energy tends to rise to the upper body, losing the natural protective function of the elbow joints for the ribs.

Both shoulders should be evenly lowered, and "dropping the shoulders" should not be mistakenly interpreted as "pressing the shoulders" and losing flexibility. When in a fixed stance, both shoulders should be relaxed and slightly forward, implying a forward relaxation of the scapulae. The mutual traction of the arm girdles naturally generates a connected, through-line sensation. This is referred to as "shoulders level and smooth, both arms linked." Such practice aids in enclosing the chest and straightening the back, enhancing the flexibility and suppleness of the shoulder joints through persistent practice.

The wrist should be relaxed and active. When in a fixed stance or when the palm is pushed forward to its endpoint, the wrist should slightly sink and exert force, with the fingers and palm slightly straightening, a process known as "settling the wrist" or "dropping the wrist." Some misunderstand "settling the wrist" and create a rigid bend in the wrist, making the forearm stiff and ineffective, similar to a tight grip. When retracting the arm, the fingers and palm gradually return to a slightly bent state, and the wrist accordingly relaxes to a straight position. Creating a rigid concave at the wrist pulse point leads to stiffness and impeded circulation, similar to an incorrect "settling the wrist."

During movement, the opening and closing transitions of the arm should follow an arc, ensuring wrist rotation and forearm (here referring to the lower arm) spiraling, making the arm's advance and retreat form spiral movements. Some Tai Chi Chuan styles emphasize: "The hands turn as if threaded," "Let the arm bone rotate to draw true strength." This approach allows for a greater variety and efficiency of force compared to straightforward arm movements and facilitates venous blood return to the heart. The downward pressure generated by dropping the shoulders and elbows, combined with the upward and forward pushing force from dropping the elbows and settling the wrists, plus the rotational force from arm muscle rotation, is one of the key factors in Tai Chi Chuan's principle of using lesser force to overcome greater force.

## 6. What Are the Requirements for the Head and Neck in Tai Chi Chuan?

In discussions of Tai Chi Chuan, various terms have been used to describe the posture of the head and neck, such as "lifting the crown," "hanging the crown," "suspension of the head," "lifting the head," "ethereal and energetic lifting," "lifting with emptiness," "straight lifting of the head," "proper alignment with suspended crown," "vertical alignment of the head and neck," "retracting the chin with an ethereal neck," "relaxed neck with suspended crown," and "leading with the head and neck." The rotation of the body is primarily determined by the brain, with state reflexes also playing a significant role. For instance, suspending a cat by its legs and dropping it shows that its head and neck twist first, subsequently flipping the body to land on its legs, demonstrating a basic physiological state reflex experiment. This experiment helps us understand the importance of "leading with the neck" in Tai Chi Chuan.

The various expressions regarding the posture of the head and neck mainly aim to achieve proper "neck leading," ensuring that head movements are correct and appropriately scaled, utilizing state reflexes for natural body coordination. It's crucial to avoid tilting or excessively leaning the head and neck, preventing neck muscle rigidity, loss of flexibility and naturalness, thereby affecting the body's flexible and complete motion and natural balance. Although ancient practitioners could not provide a scientific explanation with modern knowledge, they accumulated rich experience through long-term practice, described using terms like "lifting," "topping," "hanging," "suspending," "emptying," "releasing," and "energizing."

That is, during practice, the head should generally maintain a vertical position as if it were suspended by a rope from above. When turning the head to the side, it should rotate along the vertical axis without tilting or leaning. Head turns should coordinate with body rotation, not moving independently of the body and arms. The head and neck should gradually lead the spinal movement, ensuring the torso's rotation is unified from top to bottom.

Many misunderstand "energetic lifting" as forcibly pushing the head upwards, resulting in neck stiffness, upward flow of Qi and blood, and disruption of the body's coordination. This is similar to an interesting experiment where athletes wear a special head immobilizer and then perform movements. Restricted head movement leads to incorrect muscle tension regulation, making movements rigid and forced. Some Tai Chi Chuan texts mystify their explanations, causing misunderstandings, like boasting in the "Song of Whole Body Utilization" about "always retaining the monkey head," which refers to a simple posture of slightly tucking in the chin to protect the throat, intentionally written as "monkey head" to obscure understanding. While this helps protect the forehead and throat from strikes, overly retracting the chin can hinder natural breathing and affect coordinated and flexible movements, including natural arm extension and "sinking the Qi to the dantian." Therefore, beginners should understand that "energetic lifting" only requires a gentle upward intention; "tucking the forehead" should not be exaggerated, simply ensuring the head and neck are upright and lightly leading the body.

A correct head position involves more than avoiding left or right tilts; it maintains the cutaneous tragi (above the ear canals) and the lower orbital margins approximately level (see Illustration 1), ensuring natural head alignment and relaxed neck muscles.

Changes in head posture can alter the tension (strength) across the entire body. The reason head position changes affect whole-body muscle tension is due to the excitation of neck muscles, skin sensations, and vestibular apparatus, immediately reported to the medulla oblongata, which reflexively redistributes the body's muscle tension. Animal experiments show that removing the brain above the medulla in cats eliminates higher brain inhibition, revealing state reflexes. Adjusting the cat's head position affects limb muscle tension accordingly. Similarly, in humans, experiments show that such reflexes play a significant role in movement. For example, turning the head left increases the tension in the left arm and leg, explaining why turning the head left enhances the push in push hands; bowing the head suppresses arm extensor muscles, aiding in bending the arm; looking up strengthens arm extensor muscles, facilitating extension and force generation. Thus, to move the body lightly and flexibly, the head and neck must remain upright and lead the body's movements with relaxed and coordinated neck muscles.

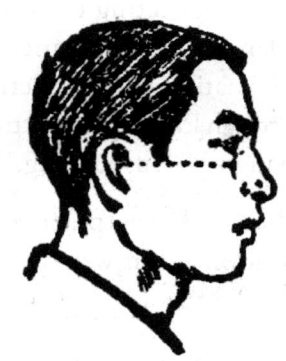

*Illustration 1*

"Lightness and agility with the head suspended" is a summary of years of practice by predecessors. It's emphasized that the head and neck should be "generally" upright, meaning the head and neck should not be rigid during practice. Aside from turning to drive torso rotation, the head and neck should slightly incline with posture changes; in push hands, more significant inclination may be needed for effective force generation. When striking with a fist or palm, the chin moves slightly forward; retracting the arm often involves more noticeable chin tucking.

Through analysis, the Baihui acupoint (where a line between the tips of the ears intersects with the midline between the front and back of the head) not only involves gentle upward tension but also changes with posture. If turning left, the head's left upper corner and Baihui lead the body; turning right, the right upper corner and Baihui lead. When tucking the chin, the force is at the fontanelle (in front of Baihui), with a gentle lift behind the ears; looking up places the force behind Baihui. Moving this way allows the head and neck to lead the body, achieving a vibrant, unified, and fluid appearance.

With proficient practice and coordination between the head, neck, and body, simply "raising the spirit" during practice corrects the head and neck posture without explicit focus, achieving the "ethereal" leading. This is akin to riding a bicycle proficiently, where foot and hand movements naturally coordinate without conscious effort.

The face should be natural, eyes naturally open, following the primary hand movements; the mouth should be lightly closed.

## 7. What requirements does Tai Chi have on the mouth?

In the practice of Tai Chi Chuan, a discipline renowned for its holistic approach to health and well-being, particular attention is paid to the nuances of the practitioner's body, including the mouth. This detailed attention supports the flow of Qi, or vital energy, and enhances the practitioner's internal harmony. Here, we delve into the specific requirements for the mouth area, which encompasses the lips, teeth, tongue, breathing, and saliva.

### Lips:

The lips should neither be tightly closed nor widely opened, but rather held in a position that feels natural and comfortable to the individual. This can mean gently closed or slightly open depending on personal comfort and physical attributes. For instance, individuals with longer lips may find it natural to keep them closed, while those with shorter lips or nasal conditions that impede breathing might slightly open their mouths. This practice is encapsulated in the ancient wisdom of maintaining a state that is "as if closed but not closed, open but not open," emphasizing a natural state where breathing is not obstructed by either extreme. Overly tight lips can hinder breathing, while wide opening is unhygienic, aesthetically displeasing, and disrupts the tranquil and deep breathing essential to Tai Chi. Moreover, inhaling cold air through a wide-open mouth can compromise health, particularly in the cold of winter, possibly leading to pharyngitis.

## Teeth:

The teeth should not be clenched but slightly parted, maintaining a relaxed state that allows for a natural gap. This relaxation extends to the masticatory muscles, aiding in the secretion of saliva.

## Tongue:

The tongue should rest naturally in the mouth or with the tip lightly touching the upper palate. Positioning it too far back can create tension. The optimal spot is where the tip naturally rises when pronouncing the sound "yi" in Mandarin. This positioning facilitates saliva flow.

## Breathing:

For details on breathing, please refer to the respective section in this book.

## Saliva:

When saliva is present, it should be swallowed regularly and not expelled. This helps prevent dryness in the mouth and throat. Recent studies both domestically and internationally have revealed that saliva contains not only amylase but also lipase, oxidase, peroxidase, hydrogen peroxide enzyme, arginine deaminase, and dehydratase. The presence of protease and coenzyme in saliva can depolymerize food, aiding in digestion and appetite enhancement. Furthermore, some recent studies suggest saliva may have anti-cancer properties, and the salivary glands might also perform endocrine functions.

These practices highlight the intricate balance and awareness cultivated in Tai Chi Chuan, where even the most seemingly minor adjustments can significantly affect the practitioner's overall energy flow and health.

## 8. What are the requirements for the chest and back in Tai Chi Chuan?

In the nuanced art of Tai Chi Chuan, the posture of the chest and back holds a place of importance, guided by the principle of "keeping the chest contained and the back lifted." This concept, often misunderstood, leads some to adopt a hunched and unattractive posture that is not only aesthetically displeasing but also detrimental to health. To address these misconceptions, clarifications such as "containing the chest does not mean collapsing it, as doing so could lead to illness" and "the most critical aspect of containing the chest and lifting the back is to avoid any inclination to slouch" are emphasized, aiming to correct the tendency towards a rounded back and caved chest. The essence of "containing the chest" is not about forcefully thrusting the chest outwards but rather about gently bringing the arms inward, allowing the chest muscles to relax without forcefully expanding the chest or holding the breath. Achieving this naturally facilitates "lifting the back," creating a posture where the spine is extended and comfortable.

The posture of "containing the chest and lifting the back" is not static but dynamically integrated into movements such as exhaling, lowering the body, and performing pushing or pressing actions. From a health perspective, everyday activities often involve using the arms in front of the body (such as writing or hoeing), offering few opportunities to open the chest. Setting aside the martial applications, naturally opening the chest during Tai Chi practice is beneficial and harmless. Therefore, during inhalation, the chest should be allowed to expand comfortably, facilitated by relaxing the shoulders, which supports abdominal breathing. Upon exhaling, the ribs and attached muscles naturally lower and relax due to gravity, reducing the chest cavity's size in a process known as "contracting the ribs and lowering the breath."

A relaxed chest facilitates smooth breathing and avoids the detrimental effects of chest tension or deliberately holding one's breath, which interrupts the natural and deep rhythm of breathing. Such tension not only hampers the lungs' capacity for renewal but also impedes the return flow of blood to the heart, particularly disadvantaging those with cardiovascular diseases. Hence, maintaining a posture of a relaxed chest and a settled abdomen is crucial for excelling in Tai Chi Chuan, enhancing overall health and the fluidity of one's practice.

## 9. Is it about "relaxed abdomen" or "engaged abdomen"? Can practicing Tai Chi Chuan lead to a big belly?

In the discourse surrounding Tai Chi Chuan, a question often arises regarding the abdominal area: should it be "relaxed" or "firm"? This question stems from traditional Tai Chi theories that mention concepts such as "relaxing the abdomen allows energy to gather into the bones," "broadening the chest with a firm abdomen," or "an empty chest with a firm abdomen," which can be perplexing. The relationship between a "relaxed abdomen" and a "firm abdomen" is dialectically unified, representing two aspects of the same principle. Only by minimizing unnecessary tension in the abdominal muscles, achieving a "relaxed abdomen," can one ensure deep, tranquil, and even breathing. This enhances abdominal breathing or diaphragmatic movement, increasing intra-abdominal pressure changes. Such dynamics act as an "internal massage" for the abdominal organs, improving blood circulation, nutrient absorption, and metabolism. This process gradually leads to a sensation of energy filling the abdomen, what is referred to as a "firm abdomen," where energy is centered in the lower abdomen (see Section 33). Hence, achieving a "relaxed abdomen" is a prerequisite for realizing a "firm abdomen," which should not be confused with forcibly tensing the abdominal muscles but rather refers to a state where the abdomen is relaxed yet filled with vibrant energy.

For beginners, it is essential to start with relaxing the abdomen, gradually progressing to the sensation of a "firm abdomen" through prolonged practice rather than hastily pursuing it. Forcing efforts can actually hinder the attainment of a "firm abdomen."

To achieve a relaxed abdomen, maintaining a calm demeanor is crucial, as well as paying attention to the posture during Tai Chi practice. For instance, the body leaning back before performing the "Lan Que Wei" (Grasping Sparrow's Tail) press movement, if done without incorporating "containing the chest and lifting the back," tucking the pelvis, and bending the hips, can lead to a backward-leaning stance, resulting in shallow, short breaths and tensed abdominal walls, which is counterproductive to relaxing the abdomen.

Concerns about practicing Tai Chi leading to a larger belly are unfounded. Tai Chi movements, such as the turning of the abdomen left and right, effectively exercise the internal and external oblique muscles, while movements like kicking can significantly strengthen the rectus abdominis. Deep and long breathing exercises, as well as the forceful movements during push hands practice, can effectively strengthen the abdominal muscles, thereby not leading to an increase in belly size.

An enlarged abdomen in some individuals is not caused by practicing Tai Chi but rather by overall body obesity, accumulation of fat in the abdominal area due to lack of physical activity or exercise, energy consumption imbalance, or metabolic and endocrine disorders. Those with a larger belly can gradually reduce its size by controlling their diet, especially by consuming less fatty food, and actively practicing Tai Chi Chuan.

# 10. Why does Tai Chi Chuan particularly emphasize the waist?

Regarding previous Tai Chi theories, we need to discard the dross and take the essence. For example, the statement "the source of intention lies in the waist" obviously exaggerates the importance of the waist, which does not conform to physiology. In fact, the central nervous system is the most important, and the generation of intention is not in the waist, but in the brain. As for the statements "always pay attention to the waist", "the waist is the axle", "practicing boxing without practicing the waist, lifelong skill will be difficult to improve", "liveliness in the waist", "from the feet to the legs to the waist must be a complete flow", "if there is no proper timing and position, the problem must be sought in the waist and legs", "the waist is like a screw, the legs are like drills", etc., are basically correct. These all indicate that the waist plays a very important role in Tai Chi movements.

How to make the waist posture correct during movement is undoubtedly one of the important issues for beginners of Tai Chi. If you do well with the three words relax, drop, and straight, the waist posture can be generally correct. Because this part is important, to explain this issue in more detail, we must first understand the normal shape of the human spine. Originally, from the embryo to full development, the development state of the spine can also explain the history of human development. The spine of a modern adult, viewed from the side, is elongated in an "S" shape (Illustration 2), with the lumbar part bending forward, while the lumbar part of an infant does not bend forward, its flat appearance is similar to that of quadrupeds. Viewed from the front, the vertebral bodies gradually enlarge from top to

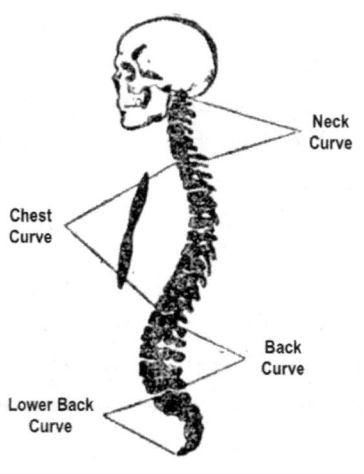

*Illustration 2*

bottom, which is different from quadrupeds. The reason why the human spine has this shape is mainly due to the upright walking posture.

Normal curvature of the spine can increase the elasticity of the spine, buffer shocks, protect the brain, and expand the volume of the thoracic and pelvic cavities to accommodate internal organs. Additionally, the internal organs of the chest and abdomen are located in front of the spine, so the forward curvature of the lumbar spine can play a certain balancing role in stabilizing the center of gravity when standing upright.

In Tai Chi theory, there are different terms for waist posture, such as bow waist, straight waist, fill waist, sit waist, collapse waist, etc. In fact, the meanings expressed by these different terms are basically consistent. From the literal meaning, these terms seem to contradict each other, but if analyzed from an anatomical perspective, it can be seen that their requirements for waist posture are essentially to reduce the forward curvature of the lumbar spine. For example, straight waist and bow waist, on the surface, these are two opposite terms, but both practices and requirements are to eliminate the forward curvature of the waist as much as possible. From an anatomical perspective, straight waist is more reasonable, while bow waist can easily be misunderstood as a bending bowing posture. However, doing a straight waist in practice does indeed have a slight backward bowing feeling in the waist. This is just an illusion of the waist straightening out. If we correctly use this "bow waist feeling", we can achieve a straight waist appearance, like filling the hollows on both sides of the spine and below the twelfth rib (this can be felt by hand), so it is also called fill waist. This is an effective method to straighten the forward curved waist. As for relax waist, sit waist, and collapse waist, they are also effective measures proposed from various angles or aspects to achieve a straight waist. In addition, dropping the buttocks or pulling the tailbone forward also mainly aims to achieve a straight waist.

Now the problem arises, since the normal curvature of the spine is a product of human upright walking, then practicing Tai Chi to straighten its curvature, restoring the waist state of quadrupeds with "tiger back and bear waist", would it not violate physiology? Indeed, if simply requiring the straightening of the waist curvature, such concerns are correct, and this is also a factor why some people cannot do the waist correctly when practicing. These people do not do the straight waist posture well because they neglect the coordination of the waist with other parts. To truly do a straight waist, besides making the waist relax, sink, and stretch, the most important links are bending the hips (also called absorbing the hips, cutting the hips, relaxing the hips, dropping the hips, or sitting the hips) and bending the knees. Bending the hips and knees is also a clever compensation method after straightening the waist, not only making the straight waist easier to do but also allowing the forward bending of the knees to replace part of the physiological requirement of the waist bend. From a biomechanical perspective, this can fully utilize the efficiency of the leg muscles. Everyone knows that most of the origin and insertion points of the waist muscles are relatively close, the muscles are shorter, the lever effect and mechanical efficiency are not significant, while the anatomical structure of the knee and hip joints is solid, the origin and insertion points of the muscles are longer, and the lever effect efficiency is strong. Of course, this method is beneficial whether in stance training or push hands, making it easier to exert force.

When bending the knees, the muscles at the back of the thighs are in a relaxed state, making the pelvis easy to move, and the hip joints very flexible, also ensuring the natural movement of the lumbosacral joints. The flexibility of the lumbosacral joints is the key to "liveliness in the waist". Therefore, in Tai Chi movements, the two legs should generally not be in a straight state, the knee joints should have some degree of bend to avoid the muscles at the back of the thighs from being tense and fixing the pelvis too rigidly, affecting the smooth transition of postures.

In daily life, if you can develop the correct method of using leg muscles, lifting heavy objects without bending the waist but using the method of bending the hips and knees, it can greatly improve work efficiency and greatly reduce waist injuries. Tai Chi has a certain effect on mastering the correct method of using leg muscles to replace bending the waist.

Another benefit of straightening the waist bend is to relax the abdominal muscles, which can provide favorable conditions for natural breathing during practice.

Besides straight waist, there are also long waist, twisting waist, or rotating waist, and the changes of emptiness and fullness in the waist. For example, in "Grasp the Sparrow's Tail" in Simplified Tai Chi, when warding off and pressing, the buttocks should drop, and the waist should have an elastic stretching upward state, which is "long waist". The focus of rolling back is on twisting the waist, and pressing combines twisting waist and long waist. When the posture is compact, straight turning can be done with simultaneous left and right rising and falling movements, that is, when the body turns left, the left waist slightly pulls up, using the right waist to support the left waist, and when turning right, the right waist slightly pulls up, using the left waist to support the right waist; but it is difficult to do this when the posture is open, beginners do not need to force it. The changes of emptiness and fullness in the waist are consistent with those in the legs: when the left leg is full, the left waist is full and the right waist is empty, and when the right leg is full, the right waist is full and the left waist is empty. One of the essences of Tai Chi is "lively waist", when advancing, retreating, or shifting steps, attention should first be paid to relaxing and sinking the waist and hips on the full leg side, making the full leg more stable and the empty leg lighter, using the full leg to send the empty leg. For example, when advancing into a bow stance, the heel of the front foot touches the ground, gradually the whole foot lands flat, then continue to advance the front knee lightly, when the knee aligns with the toe, continue to advance the hip lightly, when the bow stance is completed, the waist should be relaxed. When retreating or shifting sideways, the toes touch the ground first, then gradually bend the knee, drop the hip, and relax the waist. When the front foot hooks during the bow stance, the waist relaxes towards the heel of the front foot, making the front toe rise lightly, then hook the foot. The relaxed and lively movement of the waist has a positive functional stimulation on the spinal nerves and autonomic nerves. As the theory of traditional Chinese medicine believes, all internal organs rely on the marrow for nourishment, coupled with the coordination of diaphragm and abdominal muscle movements, this practice has a particularly positive impact on eliminating blood stasis in the internal organs and improving intestinal peristalsis function, and is especially effective in preventing and treating back pain. Most back pain is due to partial muscle spasms in the back, and the gentle movement of the waist in Tai Chi is a good method to relieve muscle spasms, promote joint flexibility, and improve blood circulation. For heavy physical labor, especially jobs that often require bending over (the most typical are bricklayers and lathe operators), regularly practicing Tai Chi is quite effective in preventing back pain. Some investigations have shown that consistently practicing Tai Chi has good effects on the shape and structure of the spine: for example, only 25.8% of a group of elderly people who regularly practice Tai Chi have spinal deformities, while it is 47.2% for the general elderly. Hunchback is a typical elderly deformity, a result of aging, and its incidence is much lower among elderly people who regularly practice Tai Chi compared to the general population. The flexibility of the spine is also better, with 77.4% of the Tai Chi group able to touch the ground with their hands when bending over, compared to 16.6% of the general elderly. The incidence of senile osteoporosis is also lower in the Tai Chi group (36.6% compared to 63.8%). Senile osteoporosis is a degenerative change due to aging, mainly because osteoblasts in bone tissue are not active, unable to produce bone protein matrix, resulting in less bone formation, more absorption, and bone becoming loose. In addition, arteriosclerosis reduces the blood supply to the bones, and reduced stomach acid in the elderly affects the absorption of calcium and phosphorus from food, all of which are causes of osteoporosis. Loose bones are prone to deformities, and joint movements become inflexible. Therefore, practicing Tai Chi also has a certain anti-aging effect.

In practicing Tai Chi, some people propose "if the opponent does not move, I do not move; if the opponent moves slightly, I move first", which is difficult for beginners to understand. In fact, this is just a specific application of the "waist and spine as the axis" in push hands, like the axle of a car or the hinge of a door or window, with very small movement, while the wheels and door panels have large movement; similarly, the movement method of the waist and spine as the axis becomes one of the foundations for moving after the opponent but arriving first.

Anatomically, the waist is the pivot of body movement. Through the various movements of the waist mentioned above, besides being closely related to the pelvis, abdomen, and lower limbs, it is also connected to the upper body. Especially the long back muscles that originate from the sacrum, lumbar vertebrae, and lumbar dorsal fascia, extending upward to the back of the neck, continuously stretching and contracting during practice, giving a feeling of continuous connection from top to bottom, with force emanating from the spine. This feeling can only be experienced on the basis of relaxation and stillness. Paying attention to the movement of the waist can also further concentrate the mind, which is one of the means to adjust the function of the nervous system and improve health.

To help beginners quickly master the waist posture, basic exercises of squatting against the wall can be used. The specific method is to stand with feet parallel, one fist apart or shoulder-width apart, heels about one foot to the length of one's thigh away from the wall. After standing well, slowly bend the knees to squat, the back and buttocks should not leave the wall, and the heels should not leave the ground. The degree of squatting increases gradually with skill growth. Long-term practice helps to straighten the waist, tuck the buttocks, and strengthen the leg power. If there is no support, repeated full squats can be done, but special attention should be paid to maintaining the relaxed waist and tucked buttocks state during squatting and standing up. Such single practice not only helps to develop a straight waist posture but also enhances leg strength, helping the elderly to walk steadily and squat and stand up freely.

## 11. What are the Tai Chi Chuan Requirements for the Buttocks and Groin Area?

Tai Chi Chuan places strict demands on the posture of the buttocks, insisting on various adjustments such as dropping, tucking, wrapping, protecting, adjusting the groin, suspending the groin, and keeping the tailbone (coccyx) aligned. These adjustments prevent the buttocks from twisting or protruding backward during movement, which can cause the natural drooping posture of the buttocks to be lost.

Some beginners, in an attempt to tuck in their buttocks, might tense their lower abdomen or forcefully pull their buttocks forward. This not only looks unattractive and stiff but also disrupts natural breathing and affects lower body stability. The correct approach involves relaxing the muscles of the buttocks and waist as much as possible, gently stretching the buttock muscles outward and downward, and then lightly pulling them forward and inward. This is akin to wrapping the pelvis with the buttock muscles, creating a sensation of securely lifting the lower abdomen with the buttocks. This action, similar to the rear counterweight of a crane, can enhance the upward lifting force of the arms. The tailbone is slightly pulled forward, aligning with the body's direction, much like a ship's rudder steering its course. This alignment not only maintains the spine's upright position but also allows the abdominal muscles to relax more easily, keeping the internal organs in their natural position for deep and comfortable breathing. It also slightly lowers the body's center of gravity, facilitating balance. However, to achieve this relaxed and inwardly tucked posture of the buttocks, bending the hips and knees is essential for pelvic flexibility. Maintaining this natural droop and slight forward tuck of the buttocks enhances the power stored in the buttocks, making it easier to transfer this force during push hands.

Tai Chi Chuan pays special attention to the strength of the waist and groin, primarily focusing on the power generated from the waist and hips. The pelvis, composed of the hip bones and the tailbone, plays a significant role as it connects the femur (thigh bone) below to the lumbar spine above. Correctly positioning the buttocks enhances flexibility and stability in the waist and legs. Therefore, the saying "rely on the hip as if it were the waist" and the advice "one hip lifts as the other drops, using highs and lows extensively, the lower body's pivot lies here, do not waste this area" emphasize the importance of hip movement. For instance, when stepping left, the left hip slightly lifts and is supported by the right hip, and vice versa for stepping right. When performing a solo posture, the hip's lifting and supporting action should be more pronounced than during stepping to achieve the state where the knee and chest draw close. In fixed postures, especially when extending the arms forward in a bow stance, coordinating a relaxed waist and dropped buttocks is crucial. If attention is also given to slightly bending the knee of the pushing leg, a deep concave can be felt at the hip joint with hand examination, which benefits pelvic flexibility and the body's balance and stability. Rotational movements, like the Roll Back force in Grasping Sparrow's Tail, require simultaneous waist and hip rotation, with the hip joint being more flexible than the waist joint, a difference that can also be felt by hand. This justifies the practice of treating the hips as the waist, where coordinating waist and hip actions leads to better results.

Regarding the groin, not only Tai Chi Chuan but also other martial arts such as Xing Yi Quan and Bagua Zhang emphasize adjustments like adjusting the groin, suspending the groin, lifting the anus, tightening the anus, lifting the perineum, and contracting the perineum. They all stress the importance of gently lifting the groin area during practice. This shows that ancient China recognized the anal and perineal regions as one of the body's weak spots. After humans evolved from quadrupedal to bipedal locomotion, the soft tissues of the perineum bore a greater load in supporting the internal organs, and the return of venous blood to the heart became more challenging. The absence of valves in the lower rectal veins makes upward blood flow even more difficult. Thus, the ancient practice of "constantly closing the earth gate" (regularly contracting the anal muscles) is invaluable, suggesting active exercises to strengthen this weak point in the human body. However, interpreting this in Tai Chi practice as forcefully lifting the anal muscles is excessive; a gentle contraction of the anal muscles suffices. With prolonged practice, the perineal area will naturally rise and fall with movement and breathing, as if suspended, hence "suspending the groin." For treating conditions like hemorrhoids, prolapse of the rectum, uterine prolapse, and vaginal wall prolapse, Tai Chi Chuan should be complemented with specific physical therapy for more significant results.

The concepts of "open groin" or "expanding the groin" mainly aim for flexible posture transitions. Specifically, by relaxing the hip joints and employing rolling steps with slight inward knee movements, the groin naturally opens, avoiding the problems of a constricted or pointed groin.

## 12. What are the requirements for Legs in Tai Chi Chuan?

The saying, "Its root is in the feet, generated through the legs," underscores that the legs are the foundation for supporting the body and the origin of force initiation. Practical experience demonstrates that the posture of the legs is crucial for ensuring correct overall body posture, stability of movements, smooth breathing, and the integrity of force (commonly known as Jin Bie). The principle of "the feet play a seventy percent role, and the hands thirty percent" highlights the significance of the legs and feet over the arms in generating force during push hands and stance work. Therefore, leg training should be given special attention.

Tai Chi Chuan also demands clear differentiation between the solid (weighted) and empty (weightless) states of the legs during advancing, retreating, and turning, ensuring stability and agility. "Differentiating between solidity and emptiness" is a key principle of Tai Chi Chuan. The leg bearing all or most of the body's weight is considered solid, and the other leg is considered empty. Only with clear differentiation between solidity and emptiness can movements be stable, agile, and transitions smooth.

The three main joints in the leg are the hip, knee, and ankle. The roles of the hip and knee can be referenced in related discussions. It is noted here that the ligaments around the hip joint are relatively tight and require a period of training to become relaxed and for the hip roots to be opened.

The requirement for leg advancement and retreat is to lift the knee before the heel, so the knee joint needs to be highly relaxed for flexible movements. Previous discussions on martial arts include the concept of "allowing freedom to the knees," where "freedom" implies a natural state. In stepping, bending the knees to a certain degree is necessary, but whether standing on one leg or bearing weight on both legs, from the beginning to the end of a posture, the knee joints should maintain a slight bend. Bending and storing energy in the legs are key for elasticity in the lower limbs and are crucial for the agility and maneuverability of body movements. Achieving this bending and storing energy allows the joints, ligaments, and surrounding muscles (such as the quadriceps) to be exercised under load. Additionally, adhering to "allowing freedom to the knees" when lifting the legs allows the knee joints and their muscular and ligamentous structures to be exercised through extension and relaxation, providing them with sufficient exercise and rest, delaying the onset of fatigue.

Traditional Chinese Medicine (TCM) believes, "The knee is the house of tendons" (from the "Inner Canon"). Indeed, the knee joint, unlike other joints in the body, relies on the protection and function of ligaments and muscles. The leg training in Tai Chi Chuan is beneficial for preventing and treating knee joint diseases.

When performing movements involving the ankle joint, such as lifting, lowering, turning in, and flaring out the toes, the actions should be slow and gentle. The heel is one of the six roots (the others being the root of the leg, arm, tailbone, ear, and neck). Whether turning on the heel or the ball of the foot has different impacts. For example, in Simplified Tai Chi Chuan, transitioning from the starting position to "Parting the Wild Horse's Mane," using the ball of the foot as the pivot for the rear leg (right leg) allows for a more agile and simple movement; if the pivot is on the heel with the ball of the foot turning inward, it is more challenging to produce an unloading force, making the outgoing rebounding force more complete.

For the aforementioned three joints, focusing only on improving their flexibility and suppleness without strengthening their robustness is incomplete. The slow transitions between the solid and empty states in the semi-squatting positions of Tai Chi Chuan effectively enhance the legs' support capacity, and the strength, suppleness, and agility of the leg muscles and joints.

Thus, there are two different views within the Tai Chi Chuan community:

1. One view holds that Tai Chi Chuan sufficiently enhances the lower body's strength, eliminating the need for additional stance training within the practice.

2. The other view suggests that additional stance training can make the three main joints of the lower body more robust.

In reality, the approach should vary from person to person. For those with patellar fatigue, arthritis, or weaker leg strength, combining stance training (standing pole) can be beneficial.

## 13. What are the Types of Stances in Tai Chi Chuan?

Step types create transient, static postures with the lower limbs forming fixed geometric shapes. Common basic step types in Tai Chi Chuan include Horse Stance, Bow Stance, T-Stance, Empty Stance, Crouching Stance, and Standing on One Leg. Step techniques refer to the methods and ways in which the lower limbs move and transition between these step types. Commonly used step techniques include Advancing Step, Retreating Step, Sideways Step, Diagonal Step, Following Step, and Adjusting Step. Step types and step techniques represent two distinct concepts: step types reflect the geometric shapes formed by the lower limbs, while step techniques reflect the methods adopted to change these geometric shapes. In other words, step types are the end result of variation, whereas step techniques are the process of change.

The execution of the basic stances is as follows:

### Horse Stance:

The Horse Stance involves standing with feet spread apart to the sides, toes pointing forward and feet parallel, avoiding inward or outward angling. The center of gravity falls between the legs, with feet apart, ranging from shoulder width to three times the foot's length. Knees are bent to make the thighs nearly parallel to the ground (or slightly more), with knees slightly turning inward but not extending beyond the toes. Shoulders relaxed, waist seated, hips dropped, creating a vertical line from the top of the head to the perineum, eyes looking straight, calm and serene, breathing naturally, chest broad with a firm abdomen (see Illustration 3), and the groin rounded (knees slightly turned in, applying slight pressure on the outside of the small toes and heels, while relaxing the hips and spreading the sides of the groin as if wrapping an object).

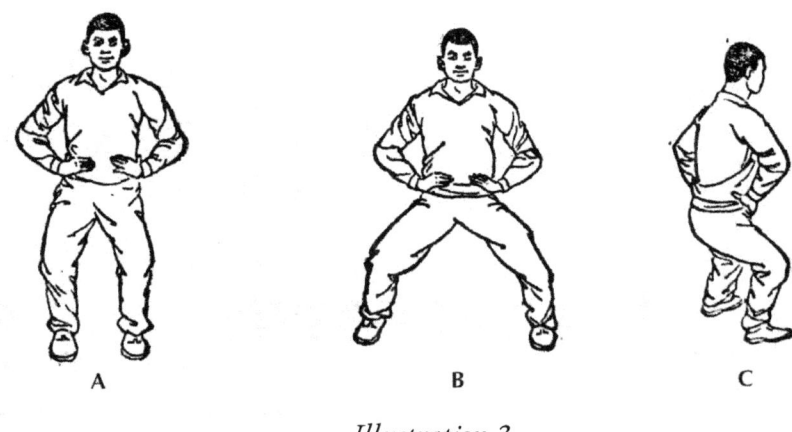

*Illustration 3*

## Bow Stance (Bow and Arrow Stance):

The Horse Stance is also known as the Bow and Arrow Stance. The front leg (bow leg) bends at the knee, which should not extend beyond the toes, with the calf not protruding beyond the heel, toes pointing forward or slightly inward. The waist is relaxed, buttocks drooping, hips dropping, bearing most of the body's weight; the back foot lightly touches the ground with the knee slightly bent, toes pointing diagonally forward or parallel to the front foot. Tai Chi Chuan frequently utilizes this stance. A left foot forward is called a "Left Bow Stance," and a right foot forward, a "Right Bow Stance." The distance between the front and back foot ranges from about a foot (measured directly) to one and a half feet (measured diagonally) or up to three times the length of one's foot. The lateral distance between the feet ranges from 10 cm to shoulder width, at a minimum, the heels should be aligned front to back (see Illustration 4). For stability and balance, aligning the outer side of the front foot in a Bow Stance with the outer side of the back foot's toe (or ball) to shoulder width is recommended.

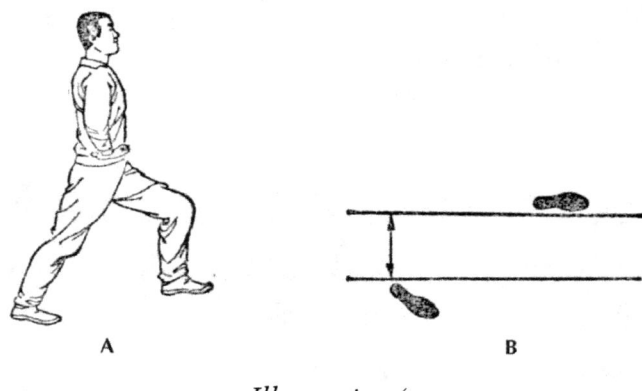

*Illustration 4*

## Empty Stance:

The back leg is bent and half-squatting, supporting the body's weight, with the front leg slightly bent, the front foot lightly touching the ground, heel slightly lifted and turned outward; or the heel gently touching the ground with the toes pointing up. Both forms are known as an Empty Stance, with a lateral distance of about 5-10 cm. Extending the left leg forward is called a "Left Empty Stance," and the right leg forward, a "Right Empty Stance" (see Illustration 5).

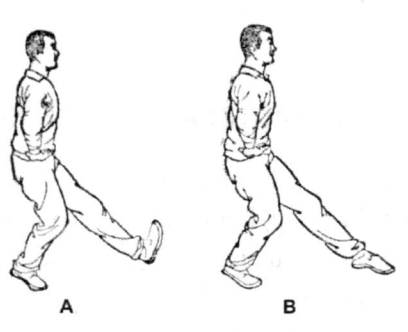

*Illustration 5*

## T-Stance (T-Step):

The T-Stance is a variation of the Empty Stance but with closer foot spacing, positioned slightly in a T-shape, one foot solidly on the ground, the other with the heel lifted and toes touching the ground. It's important to note, like the Empty Stance, that the feet should not form a perfect "T" or "□" shape but rather something in between, hence some refer to this stance as the "T-Eight Step" (see Illustration 6).

## Crouching Step:

One leg bears the weight, bending at the knee into a squat, while the other leg extends forward horizontally with the side edge of the foot pressing down,

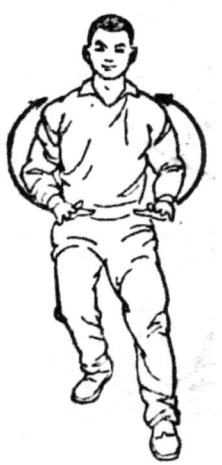

*Illustration 6*

full foot flat on the ground, knee straight, toes pointing forward at an oblique angle or a right angle (the latter being more challenging), both feet flat on the ground. The body faces sideways, looking forward. Extending the left leg straight out is called a "Left Crouching Step," and the right leg, a "Right Crouching Step." There are three different methods to practice the Crouching Step, each with its benefits. The hip higher than the knee (referring to the squatting leg's knee), especially the Crouching Step where the hip is level with the knee, because the knee joint supports the body's weight while keeping the knee from extending beyond the toes, is particularly beneficial for strengthening the knee joint's support capacity (Illustration 7A).

The Crouching Step with the hip lower than the knee, since the thigh is pressed against the calf and the knee extends beyond the toes, exerts less force on the knee joint, aiding in increased flexibility (Illustration 7B). In Chen-style Tai Chi Chuan, movements like "Snake Creeps Down" or "Spread the Brocade" require the stretching leg's calf to touch the ground, buttocks dropping while the groin lifts, and toes pointing up, offering better flexibility training for the knee and hip joints, suitable for youth practice (Illustration 7C).

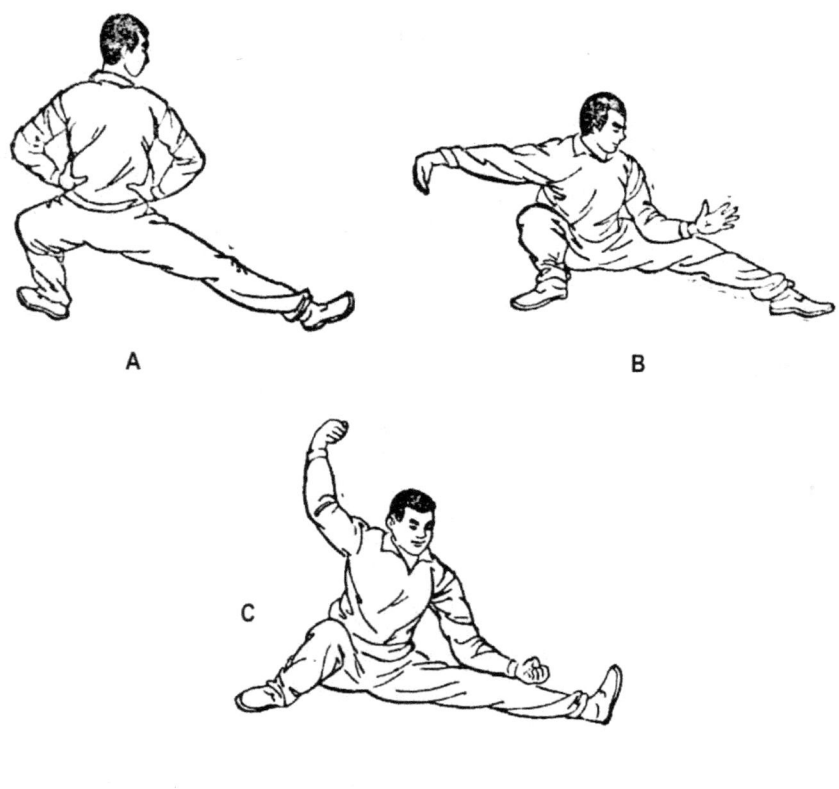

*Illustration 7*

### Standing on One Leg:

The standing leg's toes slightly point forward and outward, with the knee slightly bent; the lifted knee's toes point slightly downward and forward, ensuring the foot's arch is not tense (some Tai Chi styles advocate pointing the toes upward, primarily for striking techniques). Initially, lift the knee to navel height; with more practice, lift the knee to chest level. Standing on one leg requires the head to lead with a lifting sensation, intent focused on the lower abdomen, and using the intention to press down and sink with both the sole and heel, making standing stable(Illustration 8).

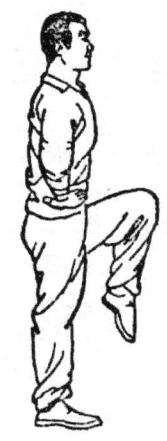

*Illustration 8*

## 14. What is the Essence of Tai Chi Chuan Footwork.

Correct footwork transformation must rely on the movement of the waist and hips. "Practicing boxing without a lively waist, lifelong skill will be difficult to improve" is a summary of many years of experience in the martial arts community of our country. If you cannot correctly use the waist and legs, movements will be stiff, coordination between upper and lower body will be difficult, and the center of gravity will not be well adjusted. It can be seen that footwork is the foundation of whole-body movement, and the movement of the waist and hips is the key to upper and lower coordination. Once these two are clarified and mastered correctly, learning boxing becomes much easier.

Tai Chi theory mentions footwork: "From the feet to the legs to the waist, it must be a complete flow; advancing and retreating, only then can you get the right timing and position; if you do not get the right timing and position, the body will be scattered and unbalanced, and the problem must be sought in the waist and legs, this applies to all directions, up and down, front and back, left and right"; "The lower part, two feet set the foundation"; "Stepping like a cat"; "Steps follow the body changes" (when the body changes, the footwork must follow); "Emptiness and fullness should be clearly distinguished, each place has its own emptiness and fullness, everywhere follows this one emptiness and one fullness"; "Emptiness is not completely without strength, fullness is not completely stiff"; "The body must be upright and comfortable", etc. These statements all explain that practicing boxing requires attention to the correct transformation of footwork and the waist and hips.

Beginners should first practice the foot positions, making them accurate. If time permits, each foot position can be practiced as stance training, and after leg strength is enhanced, then practice footwork. When practicing footwork such as advancing, retreating, stepping forward, padding step, covering step, reverse step, jumping step, leaping step, side step, following step, walking step, swinging step, and hooking step, attention should be paid to the sequence and priority of leg movements, the method and direction of foot lifting and landing, the distance between the feet when landing, and the direction the toes are pointing. The foot should lift lightly and land steadily. Generally, when advancing, the heel touches the ground first, then the whole foot slowly steps down; when retreating, the toes touch the ground first, then the whole foot slowly steps down. In the past, footwork was called the foundation (lower base or ground base) skill. When evaluating the quality of boxing practice, the first thing to look at is whether the footwork is accurate, stable, light, and smooth. When advancing and retreating, the empty leg should naturally relax and lean towards the full leg before stepping out. This is the key to maintaining an upright and comfortable body posture, and also the key to light and stable footwork.

When performing continuous bow steps forward, the body weight should be completely on the front foot, stabilizing the body, with one leg bent to support the whole body. The back leg should first lift the knee, then the heel lightly lifts off the ground, the toes drooping diagonally, then the leg gradually straightens and steps out, the heel touches the ground first, then the whole foot slowly steps down. In simplified Tai Chi, when lifting the leg to step, do not move the upper body forward together, but after the heel touches the ground first, the sole slowly steps down while the knee bends and the upper body moves forward slowly. When the sole steps down, the toes grip the ground and the lower leg feels slightly stressed, the knee is just aligned with the toes, and the center of gravity is just in the right position. This method prevents the step from being too large and allows the supporting leg to practice bearing weight for a longer time, and the stepping leg can be retracted freely. The landing point of the step not only relates to the front and back distance between the feet but also involves the lateral distance between the feet, generally about one fist to shoulder width apart, at least the heels of both feet should be aligned front and back (in a bow step, the front foot's toes point straight forward, the back foot's toes point diagonally forward, forming a T or eight-character state). The closer the heels are to a straight line, the harder it is to maintain left-right balance. If the back foot has no diagonal angle and both toes point forward, forming a straight line front to back without lateral distance, it will be unstable, often disrupting the "upright tailbone".

Except for Wu (Hao) style Tai Chi, when doing a bow step, the upper body should not lean forward, the back leg should be straight but not stiff, and should not have a noticeable bend. At the moment of exerting force, the back leg should quickly relax after straightening to maintain a state of seeming straight but not straight.

In Wu (Hao) style Tai Chi, when doing a bow step, the front and back distance between the feet is smaller, the upper body leans forward (generally, the root of the ear does not exceed the toes of the front foot), forming a diagonal straight line from the top to the heel of the back foot, with the eyes looking forward horizontally. This is called the "pillar style" (a slanted pillar used to prevent walls from collapsing). This posture makes it difficult to lean back during push hands and forms a state that makes it difficult for the opponent to attack forward, even forcing the opponent to retreat. However, when using this body method, the front and back distance between the feet should not be too large, otherwise, the opponent may take advantage of the situation to pull back, making it difficult to follow with the steps, and easy to be controlled.

When forming an empty step, the front empty leg should slightly bend the knee, paying special attention to relaxing the waist and sitting the hips, with almost all the weight on the supporting back leg; the upper body should be upright and not tilted, the tailbone root and the heel of the supporting leg should form a vertical line; the buttocks should not protrude backward.

When forming a T-step, the supporting leg should maintain a bent knee, not standing straight. Beginners often lower their body when doing a bow step, but suddenly rise when doing a T-step, making the whole boxing practice process have inconsistent body heights, reducing leg weight-bearing practice and making the movement appear floating and unstable. In Tai Chi, except for a few postures like the lower stance, seven-inch elbow, and seven-inch lean, almost every posture maintains a consistent body height. That is to say, the degree of knee bending in the supporting leg during the entire movement process should be basically the same as when starting.

When forming a crouch step, the upper body should remain as upright as possible, the feet parallel forming a straight line or the toes of the front foot and the heel of the back foot (bent knee squatting leg) forming a straight line, both feet should be fully grounded (in Chen style Tai Chi, the straight leg in the sparrow on the ground style can have the toes pointing upward), lifting the heel of the back foot or raising the outer edge of the front foot is inappropriate.

When doing a single-leg stance, beginners find it difficult to stand steadily. When transitioning from "lower stance" to "single-leg stance", the left foot should slightly turn outward, the center of gravity slowly shifts from the back right foot to the left leg, then the right foot slowly lifts, the toes naturally droop, the right hip slightly moves forward and up, aligning the right knee with the right elbow. When the right leg is in a single-leg stance, the left hip should also slightly move forward and up, aligning the left knee with the left elbow. This makes the single-leg stance easier to maintain.

# 15. What are the leg techniques of Tai Chi? How to make independent legs stand stable?

Leg techniques (□□, tuǐfǎ), commonly called foot techniques (□□, jiǎofǎ), refer to the methods of movement for the feet and legs. The main types include splitting foot (□□, fēn jiǎo), thrusting foot (□□, dēng jiǎo), kicking foot (□□, tī jiǎo), stomping foot (□□, chuài jiǎo), swinging foot (□□, bǎi jiǎo), double lifting foot (□□□, èr qǐ jiǎo), etc. According to the "Wushu Competition Rules" approved by the National Sports Commission, they are explained respectively as follows.

## Splitting (Fen Jiao):

The supporting leg is slightly bent and stable. The splitting leg is slowly raised and extended, with the foot flat and the knee slightly bent. The body should not lean backward, and both arms are held in a curved position at an equal height, fingers not higher than the head. If the arms are extended, they should not be stiff.

## Pressing (Deng Jiao):

The supporting leg is slightly bent and stable. The pressing leg is slowly raised, using the heel to press down forcefully, toes curled upwards, and the leg straightened, reaching the height of the waist or slightly higher. Both arms are held in a curved position at equal height, and the body remains upright.

## Kicking (Ti Jiao):

The supporting leg is slightly bent and stable. The kicking leg is thrust straight upward from the ground, reaching above the waist. Both arms are held in a curved position at equal height, and the body remains upright.

## Stomping (Chuai Jiao):

The supporting leg is slightly bent and stable. The stomping leg is lifted then swiftly stomped down with the heel, toes pointing up. It can also be executed with the outer side of the foot facing up for a sideways stomp, reaching above the hip. The leg must be quickly retracted after stomping. The arms move from bent to straight, and the body should not lean forward or backward (lateral tilt should not exceed 15 degrees from the vertical).

## Swinging (Bai Jiao or Bai Lian Jiao):

Swing the leg outward, ideally higher than the shoulder, with the leg straightened. The stance must be stable, hand strikes (either double or single) must be accurate, and the body kept upright. For older or weaker individuals, the leg does not need to pass over the shoulder, and strikes may target the leg instead of the foot.

## Double Lift (Er Qi Jiao):

Jump high, both feet off the ground, executing a kick and a foot slap before landing. The kicking leg should be straight, the slap loud and accurate, the body upright, and landing should be light.

For beginners practicing Tai Chi Chuan, standing on one leg during movements such as splitting or pressing can be challenging, often leading to body sway. If due to insufficient leg strength, this indicates a need for more practice or stance training to improve stability. If the technique is not mastered, it's a matter of method. Generally, following these points can help stabilize the body.

## Slowly Shift the Center of Gravity:

A common reason for instability is the failure to properly manage the center of gravity, which should be moved slowly. For example, if the left leg is the supporting leg, do not quickly lift the right leg. First, ensure the left foot is firmly planted and gradually shift all weight onto it. As the left waist and hip relax and sink, the right foot can then be slowly lifted. This approach makes it easier to maintain stability.

## Coordinate Upper Body Balance:

As a scale balances when weights on both sides are equal, so must the arms balance during movements like splitting or pressing. The arms, spread out in an arc, should be equal in angle and height, moving from up to down and outwards in an arc. This aids in maintaining stability. If the arms are spread horizontally, it can cause the body to sway. The coordination between the direction and speed of hand and foot movements, embodying the principle of "upper and lower body following each other," is crucial. This includes aligning hands with feet, elbows with knees, and shoulders with hips in an external harmony.

## Maintain a Neutral and Relaxed Body Posture:

Beginners often seek balance by incorrectly leaning or reclining the upper body while splitting or pressing, resulting in increased instability. This is often due to a fear of falling and resultant mental tension, which disrupts the natural comfort of the upper body. The correction lies in practicing "keeping the head up as if suspended from above," focusing on keeping the upper body straight and relaxed. This allows the supporting leg to be more stable.

## Keep the Supporting Leg Slightly Bent:

Not only does this lower the body's center of gravity, providing a buffer and compensation, but it's also crucial for maintaining balance. This slight bend in the joint of the supporting leg is an essential measure for stability.

## 16. What is The Practice and Significance of Stance Training in Tai Chi Chuan?

Stance training, also known as Zhan Zhuang or "standing like a post," is a crucial foundational practice in martial arts. The saying in the martial arts community, "Practicing martial arts without stance training is like building a house without pillars," vividly underscores the importance of stance work. Practicing Tai Chi without stance training is akin to constructing a grand timber structure without any supporting pillars. Common stance practices in Tai Chi Chuan include the Hun Yuan stance and the Jia Ma stance. The Hun Yuan stance is suitable for the elderly, the weak, or those with chronic illnesses. Of course, it is also beneficial for healthy individuals as a form of health maintenance or fundamental practice. However, younger and stronger individuals may find quicker progress with the Jia Ma stance.

### Hun Yuan Stance

Stand with feet parallel and shoulder-width apart, knees slightly bent in a squatting position, head level, neck straight, spine upright, and the upper body perpendicular to the ground. Relax the shoulders, waist, and hips. Raise both arms to shoulder height, with elbows slightly lower than the shoulders, embracing a large tree; fingers of both hands are spread and slightly bent as if holding a ball, with palms facing each other about a foot apart. Eyes are naturally open, gazing at a fixed point in the distance, with breathing natural (see Illustration 9).

Initially, one might only manage a few minutes, gradually increasing to 20-40 minutes. Those in better health can adopt a lower posture. Generally, after two weeks of practice, one may start to feel soreness, swelling, or pain in the legs within the first few minutes of stance training, sometimes accompanied by slight muscular tremors detectable only through close observation or touch. Continuing the stance may lead to more noticeable shaking, with the thigh muscles exhibiting rhythmic tremors and the whole body gently vibrating. Over time, as muscular endurance and control improve, the shaking may subside to very fine tremors or stop altogether. If one continues, the cycle of tremors may resume. After completing the stance, performing simple exercises to relax the leg muscles, such as squatting a few times, jumping in place, or taking a short walk, can create a warm and relaxed feeling in the legs. Those who are frail should adopt a higher stance and stop when they feel fine tremors in their thigh muscles.

In essence, stance training is a form of isometric exercise, though stillness is relative. Unlike inanimate objects, the human center of gravity constantly shifts with blood circulation, breathing, and digestion, causing internal bodily shifts that affect overall balance. Breathing, in particular, significantly impacts posture. Thus, while practicing stance training, the body's center of gravity continually moves slightly within a certain range (approximately 1.5 to 2 cm in diameter). Therefore, some individuals with a keen sense of awareness may experience sensations such as "a tree swaying in the wind," "drifting wood in water," "exhaling like a descending wild goose, inhaling as if taking flight," "light inhale, heavy exhale," and "standing firm as a mountain, moving with ease." However, those without these sensations should not intentionally pursue them, and those who experience them should not overly encourage them.

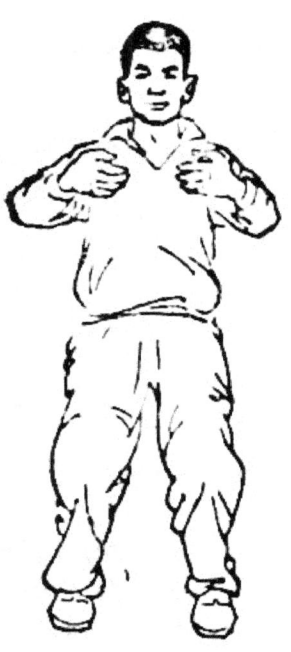

*Illustration 9*

Now, the following verse is introduced as follows:

*Relax the shoulders, loosen the hips, the value lies in a spacious waist,*
*In movement, find stillness, for the best effects to embrace.*
*Breathing in and out naturally, therein lies the wonder shown,*
*Like a tree swaying in the wind, branches moving, gracefully blown.*
*With the upper body light, and the lower firm, the feet grip the earth,*
*Throughout the body, always feel as light as a feather, in constant rebirth.*

## Horse-Clamping Stance (Jia Ma Zhuang)

Stand with your feet positioned in an inverted "V" shape, knees drawn inward, the angle of knee and hip flexion smaller than that of the Hun Yuan stance, meaning the posture is lower, but otherwise largely similar to the Hun Yuan stance. The verse for this stance is as follows:

*In the Horse-Clamping form, feet grip the ground, head touches the sky.*
*Hollow the chest, sink the breath low, elbows droop, shoulders let lie.*
*Ten fingers suspended in air, tips facing tips of the brows.*
*Inhale with self-awareness, increase gently, not reducing.*
*Stand without exerting too much, benefits come with time and touch.*

The significance of stance training primarily lies in increasing the strength of the lower limbs, strengthening the knee and ankle joints, stabilizing the lower body, and aiding in mastering relaxation and breath control during Tai Chi practice. It also has a therapeutic effect on certain conditions, such as the Horse-Clamping Stance benefiting patellar strain, and the Hun Yuan Stance having a preventive and therapeutic effect on hypertension. Some worry that stance training might stiffen the muscles. However, if relaxation exercises are performed after practice, the muscles will not only avoid becoming stiff but will also become more dynamic, flexible, and quick. Ancient practitioners also pointed out: "To achieve the marvelous utility of martial techniques, one must start with stance training to transform the weak into strong, the clumsy into agile." This has not only been confirmed by years of experience in the martial arts community but has also shown positive effects in the foundational training of other sports. For example, the medical team of the Fuzhou volleyball team observed that the trembling experienced during stance training is due to the continuous cycle of tension and relaxation in the muscle fibers, rather than a constant state of tension. Therefore, those who undergo stance training appear particularly agile and explosive, without any risk of muscle stiffening.

Additionally, practice and some scientific experiments have proven that stance training is an active method to eliminate fatigue and prevent it. Experiments have shown that isometric exercises after fatiguing dynamic work is an effective rest method. This indicates that the negative induction of the intensely excited cortical nerve cells during stance training can deepen the recovery process of work capacity.

It was also found that to improve the function of unfatigued muscles, performing isometric work on other muscle groups before the (unfatigued) muscle works can utilize isometric exercises. This phenomenon is known as "the prevention method of fatigue." The physiological mechanism of this phenomenon shows that excitement can spread from the nerve cells executing isometric tension to the motor analyzer. Hence, stance training not only strengthens the physique but is also an effective way to enhance work capacity.

## 17. What are the main techniques of Tai Chi?

In the realm of Tai Chi Chuan, a martial art that emphasizes internal strength, fluidity, and the harmonious balance of opposing forces, the mastery of hand techniques forms the cornerstone of practice. The primary hand techniques, embodying both the philosophy and physical embodiment of Tai Chi Chuan, are categorized into eight distinct movements: Ward Off, Roll Back, Press, Push, Pluck, Split, Elbow, and Shoulder. These movements, intrinsically linked to the natural world, reflect the ebb and flow of energy, the interplay between softness and strength, and the strategic redirection of force.

## Ward Off (Peng):

This technique, at its core, is about creating an upward and outward elastic force, akin to an encompassing wall, regardless of the action undertaken. In a narrower sense, it involves lifting upwards against an opponent's force, preventing it from descending, effectively neutralizing it.

## Roll Back (Lu):

Roll Back is the art of yielding; when an opponent pushes or squeezes, one responds by moving backward and downward, guiding the opponent's force in a way that causes them to stumble forward and lose their balance.

## Press (Ji):

In the context of engagement, Press involves adhering to the opponent with the hand or arm, immobilizing them momentarily before expelling them forcefully.

## Push (An):

During engagement, if an opponent attempts to press, one counters with a downward pressing motion to disrupt their force. This technique also includes the method of pressing forward.

## Pluck (Cai):

Pluck involves seizing the opponent's wrist or elbow and pulling downward, taking advantage of their forward momentum to unbalance and control them. A practitioner adept in Pluck can neutralize and counter any force.

## Split (Lie):

Split refers to the act of twisting and turning, dissolving the opponent's force and redirecting it to gain a strategic advantage, often leading to a position where lesser force can overcome greater resistance.

## Elbow (Zhou):

The use of the elbow to advance into the opponent's space, striking with precision and power.

## Shoulder (Kao):

Shoulder entails using the shoulder or back in a variety of ways—shaking, bouncing, bumping, striking—to launch an attack, particularly when in close proximity to the opponent, capitalizing on the most opportune moment.

The interpretation of these eight methods has varied among practitioners throughout history. To provide clarity and insight, the following verse offers a synthesis of these concepts, emphasizing the essential principles underlying Tai Chi Chuan's hand techniques:

***What is the meaning of 'Warding Off'?*** *It is akin to a boat pressing against the water. Begin by solidifying the energy in the lower abdomen, followed by suspending the head as if hanging from above.* ***The body acts like a spring,*** *its opening and closing maintaining a definite rhythm. No matter the strength of your body, buoyancy is not difficult to achieve.*

***What is the meaning of 'Rolling Back'?*** *It is to guide and lead forward. Follow the incoming force, agile and spirited, without losing your natural ability to keep balance.* ***When force exhausts, naturally it empties,***

*allowing strikes to flow as they will. The center of gravity maintains itself; do not let others take advantage.*

**What is the meaning of 'Pressing'?** *It involves dual aspects when applied. A direct, simple intention, engaging within the dynamics of movement.* **An indirect reaction force,** *like a ball rebounding off a wall. Or like coins striking a drum, producing a crisp and resonant sound.*

**What is the meaning of 'Pushing'?** *It operates like water flows. Within softness resides firm strength, and the rush of rapid currents is hard to oppose.* **When meeting heights, it swells;** *when finding depressions, it dives. Waves rise and fall, and where there is an opening, it fails not to enter.*

**What is the meaning of 'Plucking'?** *It is like the balance in wielding a weight. Regardless of the magnitude of the force, one weighs its lightness and heaviness afterward.* **A shift of merely four ounces** *can weigh against a thousand pounds. If you ask of the principle, it is the function of the lever.*

**What is the meaning of 'Splitting'?** *An example of the force is as follows. Like a spinning wheel, if you throw an object on top, the spinning wheel will throw it far away. The rapid flow becomes like a vortex, the curl of a wave like a screw thread. Like a fallen leaf on the surface, it is taken to the depths below.*

**What is the meaning of 'Elbowing'?** *The method comprises five elements. Dividing yin and yang, upper and lower, one must clearly manage the real and the empty.* **The posture like lotus flowers cannot be opposed;** *if opposed, the strike is even fiercer. Once the six energies are integrated, their application becomes boundless.*

**What is the meaning of 'Shouldering'?** *The technique divides between the shoulder and the back. The diagonal flying posture uses the shoulder, within which the back still plays a part.* **Once an opportunity arises,** *it thunders like pounding a pestle. Pay careful attention to maintaining the center; losing it renders the effort futile.*

To sum up, the frequently used techniques in Tai Chi Chuan are Warding Off, Rolling Back, Pressing, Pushing, Plucking, Lifting, Elbowing, and Shouldering. Among these eight techniques, the first four are more critical, with Warding Off being the most essential. Not one of these techniques should lose the resilience of the Warding Off energy. Moreover, Warding Off is the key to overcoming greater strength with lesser force. For example, if one pushes horizontally with one hand against another's chest and the opponent is stronger, pushing might not move them. However, if at that moment one sinks the shoulders and drops the elbows, applying a resilient Warding Off energy forward and upward, the opponent often becomes unstable, even if they adopt a stable stance. If Rolling Back loses the inherent resilience of Warding Off, it is often exploited by the opponent and pushed out. When Pressing directly forward, it also often fails to move the opponent unless one adds an upward twisting of the forearm, enhancing the effect of lesser force overcoming greater strength.

Some experienced practitioners have summarized the techniques of Tai Chi Chuan through their practice of forms and push hands: In Warding Off, the arms must support; in Rolling Back, the palm must be light; in Pressing, the back of the hand must be horizontal; in Pushing, the arch of the waist must attack; in Plucking, the fingers must be solid; objects between the arms must be tight; in Elbowing, the bent action must thrust; in Shouldering, the shoulder peaks must burst. The interplay of all techniques contains the essence; skillful application comes from mastery. Though these interpretations are not comprehensive and perfect, they essentially capture the primary conflict in 'Warding Off' and the main points of each technique, serving as a reference for beginners.

The explanations of these techniques are meant to aid beginners in understanding, yet with dedicated practice, the variations are numerous. Like Warding Off, there can be straight suppression, lateral embracing, upper covering, lower poking, adhering to the opponent's arm or hand, and changing directions at any moment, always ensuring the opponent has no point of leverage on oneself. When the opponent presents an opportunity, immediately change direction but keep adhering without losing contact—this is known as maintaining the Warding Off energy. Rolling Back can be upward, downward, or level; Pressing can be direct, indirect, with the addition of the elbow, folded and pressed, or flipped up or down, all depending on the specific situation at the time. Pushing varies immensely: lightly and advancing, heavily and advancing, left heavy right empty and advancing, left empty right heavy and advancing, both hands opening and pushing, both hands closing and pushing, among others, too numerous to enumerate.

# 18. How to pay attention to your eyes when practicing Tai Chi Chuan?

## On the Importance of Eye Movement in Tai Chi Chuan

In the art of Tai Chi Chuan, "hands, eyes, body, method, and steps" form the quintessence of practice, representing five pillars of training focus. It has come to our understanding that placing emphasis on the cultivation of eye movement not only exercises the ocular muscles through their relaxation and contraction but also enhances local blood circulation. As blood flow and metabolic activities intensify, the nourishment delivered to the eyes increases, gradually augmenting their function. Furthermore, the concentration of one's gaze aids in centering the spirit, maintaining mental clarity, and elevating the efficacy of movement.

## How Should One Focus One's Gaze?

During each movement, there typically is a hand designated for offense and another for defense. Practitioners should direct their gaze towards the advancing hand, essentially the one positioned more forwardly. For instance, in executing the "Single Whip" move, one should focus on the left hand; during the "Needle at Sea Bottom," the attention shifts to the right hand; and in performing "Cloud Hands," the gaze alternates between the left and right hands as they rotate upwards.

Generally speaking, the gaze follows the primary offensive hand's motion, embodying the principle of "eyes follow the hand; steps follow the body." In stationary poses, the gaze extends forward from the tips of the index or middle finger. This practice not only trains the eye muscles but also helps alleviate fatigue. Alongside the primary offensive hand's movement, the gaze should be lively and spirited, encompassing all directions—up, down, left, right—without becoming fixed or skewed, nor should one adopt an intentionally furrowed or glaring expression. Eyes ought to be naturally open, embodying "authority without aggression," reflecting a demeanor that is calm, expansive, vivacious, yet serious. The methods discussed prioritize fitness, advocating for the practice where the gaze accompanies the hand. Some argue for leading with the gaze, suggesting that the eyes should guide the hand. Historical discourse on martial arts also supports the precedence of the gaze, indicating the need for further exploration into these practices.

## Adaptations for Individuals with Health Conditions

For those who are frail, suffer from dizziness, or have severe nervous system debilitation, practicing with the gaze following the hand might induce discomfort. In such cases, adopting an approach of "eyes as if lowering a curtain," appearing neither fully open nor closed, can be beneficial. This method aids in enhancing the sensation of internal energy flow, assists beginners in memorizing movements and their nuances, and fosters introspection. Additionally, it serves as a training for vestibular function. Normally, visual supervision aids in maintaining balance due to the intricate connection between visual analyzers and the brain's cortex, which coordinates muscle movement. Therefore, practicing Tai Chi with eyes closed can positively impact balance and is especially beneficial for those with vestibular dysfunction. Thus, tailoring the practice to individual needs, allowing for a gaze that is neither fully open nor closed, is both feasible and beneficial.

## 19. What are the Body Methods in Tai Chi Chuan.

What is "Central Equilibrium and Relaxed Posture"?

The concept of body method in Tai Chi Chuan encompasses two interpretations: one refers to the posture of the torso, and the other to the movements of the entire body, including the limbs. Tai Chi Chuan delineates ten essential body methods:

1. Han Xiong (Containing the Chest)

2. Ba Bei (Extending the Back)

3. Guo Dang (Rounding the Groin)

4. Hu Zhun (Protecting the Vital Organs)

5. Ti Ding (Lifting the Crown of the Head)

6. Diao Dang (Suspending the Groin)

7. Song Jian (Relaxing the Shoulders)

8. Chen Zhou (Sinking the Elbows)

9. Shan Zhan (Evading and Countering)

10. Teng Nuo (Nimble Stepping).

These ten body methods articulate key principles regarding posture and its transformative processes. Some of these methods have been elucidated in previous discussions and will not be reiterated here. Instead, we will briefly explore "evading and countering," "nimble stepping," "protecting the vital organs," and provide a concise explanation of the principle of "Central Equilibrium and Relaxed Posture."

"Evading and countering" signifies not only agility and swiftness but also encompasses the strategy of evading the opponent's fierce momentum, simultaneously positioning oneself for a counterattack.

The notion of attack and defense in Tai Chi Chuan is not rigidly separated. A purely defensive stance awaiting an opportunity to attack, or an offensive move that lacks defensive capability, represents a unilateral application of martial strategy, failing to recognize the dialectical relationship between offense and defense. Tai Chi Chuan's method of "evading and countering" brilliantly embodies the superiority of defense within offense and vice versa, offering much greater flexibility than mere attack or defense.

It is said, "What is to evade, what is to advance? To advance is to evade; to evade is to advance. There is no need to look far." This further elucidates the relationship between evasion and advancement, defense and offense. The actions of evading and countering are unified and should not be distinctly separated.

In push hands, the body faces the opponent either directly or sideways. The transition from facing directly to sideways, or vice versa, is chiefly accomplished through twisting of the waist and hips or concurrent stepping, facilitating the actions of evading or advancing. While the ten body methods do not explicitly mention the waist and hips, the ability to perform "evading and countering" relies on the agility and flexibility of the waist and legs. In other words, "evading and countering" is a method of minimal and rapid body rotation to deflect and exploit the opponent's force, turning it into a disadvantage and swiftly countering with elastic energy. Its hallmark is avoiding direct confrontation with incoming force, appearing to make contact without really doing so, and swiftly transitioning from passive to active, using minimal effort to overcome greater force.

"Nimble stepping" refers to the dynamic and agile shifts in body posture and footwork, embodying elastic energy in stance adjustments or push hands, invigorating the spirit, and ensuring the upper and lower limbs maintain their energy during transitions between substantial and insubstantial. Special attention is required for the forearms to retain their energy.

Relaxing the shoulders and sinking the elbows facilitate the nimbleness of the forearms. The insubstantial leg suggests a mutual attraction with the torso, whereas the substantial leg does not imply full rigidity but is energetically engaged, supporting the entire body with an uplifting intent in the lower legs.

During stance adjustments or push hands, movements must incorporate lightness and agility even when slow. Slowness can transform into speed, and stability lays the foundation for agility. This underscores the significance of the body methods of "evading and countering" and "nimble stepping" to avoid sluggishness. Thus, Tai Chi Chuan does not solely advocate for slowness at the expense of agility; rather, it requires the mastery of both "evading and countering" and "nimble stepping" in body and footwork.

"Protecting the vital organs" involves a slight contraction of the flanks, adopting a posture of drawing in and combining forward movements, facilitating a relaxed and quick internal feeling. This should not result in intentional compression of the chest but rather a natural downward and forward curving of the ribcage during exhalation. Additionally, "sinking the elbows" also supports "protecting the vital organs." The term might seem esoteric, thus "protecting the chest" might be more comprehensible.

Central Equilibrium and Relaxed Posture refers to maintaining a natural and extended posture of the torso during practice, upright and stable (occasionally leaning forward or backward in some Tai Chi styles). This principle mandates the avoidance of protrusions or indentations, ensuring joints remain flexible, and directions of waist, legs, or foot placements are appropriate, preventing discomfort and unnatural feelings, in line with the requirements of Central Equilibrium and Relaxed Posture. Practicing Tai Chi necessitates relaxation of the body's muscles and joints beyond necessary tension, allowing for chest expansion and lung relaxation, thus facilitating the circulation of Qi and blood. Achieving an insubstantial leading with the head and maintaining central alignment prevents the torso from leaning forwards, backwards, or tilting sideways. Otherwise, movements will not exhibit Central Equilibrium and Relaxed Posture, affecting natural breathing, balance, and making one susceptible to being controlled during push hands.

The overarching requirement of body method is an upright posture, exuding a demeanor of centrality, openness, strictness, and extension.

## 20. Why does Tai Chi Chuan practice place special emphasis on relaxation?

The relaxation demanded by Tai Chi Chuan requires not only physical loosening but also a mental state of ease. It's crucial to understand that this form of relaxation refers to a natural, comfortable state, not to a point of laxity where the spirit wanes, muscles become so slack that one can hardly lift their head, or the wrists dare not be straightened. The correct approach involves relaxing all parts of the body except those that must remain tense.

Relaxation and tension exist in a dialectical relationship, complementing and deriving from each other. Human movement is primarily facilitated through the contraction (tension) and relaxation of muscles, which in turn, move the skeleton. These muscles can broadly be categorized into flexors and extensors. Flexors act in opposition to extensors, and vice versa. For instance, making a fist might seem like a tensing action as the flexor muscles contract, but this also necessitates the relaxation of the extensor muscles. People with severe burns on the back of their hands cannot make a fist because the scarring of the extensor muscles impedes their ability to relax and coordinate with the flexors. The same principle applies to practicing Tai Chi Chuan; without properly balancing relaxation and tension, achieving the correct posture and precise movements becomes challenging. Tai Chi Chuan movements demand harmonious and natural coordination, resembling the continuous, seamless flow of a silkworm spinning silk, clouds drifting across the sky, or pearls rolling smoothly on a plate, integrating changes between left and right, front and back, and between the substantial and insubstantial. Without a degree of tension, reaching these advanced levels of skill is impossible.

So, why is relaxation particularly emphasized in Tai Chi Chuan?

1. In work, exercise, and wakefulness, the spirit and body inadvertently lean towards a state of tension. This is especially true for beginners of Tai Chi Chuan, whose bodily movements, despite involving contraction and relaxation, tension and looseness, are predominantly tense with less relaxation. Relaxation is hard to train, whereas tension comes easily. In teaching Tai Chi, instructors often remind students "not to exert force," but it typically takes repeated practice to eliminate stiffness. Furthermore, as soon as the movements become slightly more challenging, stiffness reappears unconsciously. This, in fact, is a natural phenomenon hard to avoid with progress; each step forward involves overcoming "stiffness." Once stiffness is eliminated, movements become smooth and natural, leading to better training outcomes. The "delight in liveliness" mentioned in previous discussions on Tai Chi refers to the ongoing effort to overcome "stiffness," achieving a harmonious, comfortable feeling of coordination and relaxation throughout the body's joints and muscles.

2. For some patients, especially those suffering from chronic conditions like neurasthenia or hypertension, the spirit often remains in a pathologically tense state, even resting in unnecessarily tense postures such as clenching the teeth, shrugging the shoulders, or making fists. Conscious relaxation is a potent method for eliminating such pathological tension.

3. Relaxation serves as a form of rest against tension, an effective way to reduce fatigue and conserve energy. Engaging in muscle relaxation activities after physical labor or strength training helps to quickly restore the excitability of the neuromuscular system. This is one reason why practicing Tai Chi during breaks or after work can more effectively alleviate fatigue and restore energy than static rest.

4. In martial arts, there's a saying: "Better to lengthen a tendon by a

centimeter than to lengthen a muscle by an inch." The "lengthening" mentioned here results from relaxation, enhancing joint flexibility. Long-term Tai Chi practitioners often have slightly longer arms when extended, with a noticeable deep cavity at the shoulder socket, a result of continuous practice of relaxing the shoulders (sinking the shoulders), dropping the elbows, containing the chest, and extending the back.

5. The force used in Tai Chi movements, primarily consisting of warding off, rolling back, pressing, pushing, plucking, rending, elbowing, and leaning, hinges on warding off force, or elastic force. The saying "steel that has been forged a hundred times becomes as soft as silk" illustrates that only after extended practice can one achieve the combination of hardness and softness, elasticity in muscles. Indeed, the quality of muscle largely depends on its elasticity, and emphasizing relaxation in practice aids in enhancing muscle elasticity.

6. In some Tai Chi forms that combine fast and slow movements and require speed, relaxation is key to achieving swiftness. A punch thrown with a tightly clenched fist is not as fast as one from a relaxed hand because clenching the fist tenses the arm muscles, as if numerous small ropes are pulling and hindering the arm's motion. Thus, the correct technique involves only clenching the fist rapidly at the moment the punch reaches its target.

7. During physical activity, the body consumes more energy, necessitating the circulatory system to deliver more nutrients and oxygen while removing carbon dioxide and metabolic products. Relaxation during practice significantly increases the number of open capillaries within the muscles, promoting unobstructed blood flow. This is particularly important for areas like joints and tendons where blood vessels are sparse. Especially, the return of venous blood (notably from the lower limbs) to the heart is mainly facilitated by the rhythmic compression caused by muscle contraction and joint extension. Tai Chi's emphasis on relaxation,

coupled with movements that often trace arcs and involve spiraling limb rotations, further aids in promoting venous return, much like twisting a moist towel is more effective than simple squeezing. Additionally, muscle relaxation can reflexively induce vascular relaxation, leading to a decrease in blood pressure, thus it's crucial for individuals with hypertension to pay special attention to relaxation during practice.

8. In push hands, a skilled practitioner's arms are not only flexible but also feel significantly heavy, as if filled with mercury – heavy yet fluid, a result of relaxed joints and muscles. When lifting the arm of someone deeply asleep, it feels notably heavy due to the natural relaxation and heaviness absent of conscious control.

For those struggling with relaxation during long-term practice, the following method may help: begin in a preparatory stance with feet parallel and shoulder-width apart, letting all body joints naturally sink downwards with gravity, standing as though a bamboo pole that sways at the slightest external force. When raising the arms during the commencement form, use only the minimal necessary force to lift the arms, letting them dangle and relax over the upper limbs. Applying this principle to other postures as well can aid in mastering relaxation.

## 21. How to understand the relationship between movement and stillness in Tai Chi?

In the mid-Warring States period, the renowned military strategist Sun Bin articulated, "Static action is a marvel of movement," and "Silence in demeanor is also a form of movement." In the seventeenth century, Wang Fuzhi, a key thinker in primitive materialism and dialectics, proposed, "The static encompasses movement; it does not equate to immobility. To be static is to contain movement, and movement never abandons stillness." Lenin, a great revolutionary teacher, profoundly noted, "Movement is the unity of continuity and discontinuity in time and space." (Summary of Hegel's Lectures on the Philosophy of History, Collected Works of

Lenin, Volume 38, p. 283.) The great leader and teacher Chairman Mao insightfully stated, "In watching a film, the characters on the screen appear to be constantly moving. However, if one examines the film strip, each frame is static... The world operates on such dialectics: there is movement and there is stillness, with neither pure stillness nor pure movement existing in isolation. Movement is absolute, while stillness is temporary and conditional." (Speech at the Second Plenary Session of the Eighth Central Committee of the Communist Party of China, Selected Works of Mao Zedong, Volume 5, p. 313.) Dialectical materialism acknowledges the eternal, absolute movement of matter, which contains various relative states of rest, affirming that movement is a form of material existence without denying the presence of static states in the material world. The static state is not absolute but relative, merely a specific form of material movement. Recognizing static states does not negate the absoluteness of material movement. Previous Tai Chi Chuan theories that include "motion within stillness and stillness within motion," "seeing motion as stillness," "seeing stillness as motion," and "being still amidst motion," accurately expound the dialectical unity of motion and stillness, embodying the essence of dialectical thought, opposing metaphysics and the notion of absolute stillness. Exaggerating stillness, confusing ends with means, and making stillness the ultimate goal of practice leads to erroneous paths, entangling oneself in idealism and metaphysics.

The stillness referred to in Tai Chi Chuan denotes an all-encompassing motion where every part of the body is in movement, yet there exists a relative state of stillness. For instance, when stepping forward, the supporting foot remains relatively still compared to the moving foot. On another level, it refers to the slow movements of Tai Chi Chuan, appearing both dynamic and static. However, it primarily pertains to a mental state. Stillness is not an absence of thought, nor does it advocate for practitioners to be drowsy with eyes closed. On the contrary, stillness emphasizes engaging in practice with a composed, undistracted mind, focusing intently on the movements. In other words, stillness demands concentration, a calm, cool, collected approach following the steps and requirements of practice, earnestly training the body for the revolution, ensuring movements remain steady, gentle, and correct without stiffness, breathing naturally and effortlessly. Thus, stillness serves to enhance and regulate movement.

The dialectical unity of movement and stillness benefits the regulatory functions of excitation and inhibition within the cerebral cortex. Practicing Tai Chi induces excitation in certain areas of the cerebral cortex, transforming the excitatory state caused by thinking or single-tasking in other areas into an inhibitory state, thereby swiftly alleviating fatigue. Persistent practice can gradually break the vicious cycle of disease in the brain, offering therapeutic effects, particularly effective for neurasthenia.

## 22. What is The Relationship and Synergistic Effect of Relaxation and Stillness?

In the realm of movement, the concepts of dynamism and stillness, relaxation and tension, exist both in opposition and in unity. As the great leader Chairman Mao has taught us, "The interdependence and struggle of contradictory aspects present in all things determine their life and propel their development. There is no thing without contradiction; without contradiction, there is no world." (On Contradiction, Selected Works of Mao Zedong, p. 280) Within this framework, stillness and relaxation exert a mutual influence, enhancing and promoting each other.

1. Mental and muscular relaxation can prevent unnecessary tension, leading to reduced stimulation of the brain. This not only allows the brain to rest and the mental state to become more tranquil but also facilitates the adjustment and training of the central nervous system's functions.

2. Stillness is a necessary condition for relaxation. If the mind is troubled and restless, achieving a state of relaxed naturalness becomes impossible. Tai Chi Chuan emphasizes "coordinated movement" and "harmony between upper and lower body parts," where a calm central nervous system plays a crucial role in commanding movements, significantly aiding in the rapid acquisition of coor-

dination.

3. Tai Chi Chuan practice stresses the importance of a stable lower stance and a light and agile upper body, achievable only in a state of relaxation and stillness. This ensures the lower part of the body is solid and full, avoiding the pitfalls of top-heaviness, light-footedness, and unstable stances.

4. Stillness and relaxation are also key to training acute sensory perception. Previous discussions on martial arts have mentioned the phrase "unable to bear the weight of a feather, nor dislodge a crawling insect," a metaphor describing the sensitivity of response honed through long-term practice. However, this statement has been the subject of much debate. Some view it as an arcane expression, impossible or mystical and thus incomprehensible. Others have used it to mystify, claiming such sensitivity is only achievable by uniquely gifted "geniuses." In reality, this level of sensitivity is developed through prolonged attention to relaxation and stillness in practice and push hands, devoid of any mystery. With long-term practice, it is a technical state accessible to the average person, mirroring the insights shared by Xu Yinsheng in his article "On Playing Table Tennis." He noted, "One can immediately feel any dirt or sweat on the ball during play." Is it not possible, then, to detect an insect landing on one's skin?!

## 23. What does "Qi" refer to, and does it offer any benefits?

Some practitioners of Tai Chi Chuan report sensing Qi circulating within their bodies. This concept has been widely discussed in ancient martial arts texts, with phrases like "Qi moves like a stream of nine bends, reaching everywhere subtly," "Qi should surge," "Qi follows the body seamlessly without slipping," and "Qi sinks to the Dantian." What exactly is Qi? Opinions vary: some interpret Qi as breath, others as spirit or intent, while some believe in the existence of "Qi meridians" distinct from blood vessels, viewing Qi as a mystical essence of the cosmos flowing within us. The plethora of interpretations makes the concept of Qi complex and sometimes confusing, necessitating a clear analysis to dispel ambiguities and mystical notions.

Breath can only occur within the lungs and cannot reach the abdominal cavity or other parts of the limbs. If Qi is equated with intent or spirit, this does not explain sensations like numbness, heat, or swelling associated with Qi. Therefore, we should distinguish between breath, spirit, or "intent" in our discussion.

Patients undergoing acupuncture sometimes experience specific sensations, such as numbness, heat, or swelling, referred to as "De Qi" in ancient texts. The sensation of Qi during Tai Chi practice, similar to "De Qi" in acupuncture, also manifests as numbness, heat, swelling, or the feeling of ants crawling on the skin. What are these sensations? They result from the excitation impulses (biological electrical pulses) generated when the body's nerve endings and various receptors receive internal and external stimuli, transmitted along the afferent nerves to the cerebral cortex. Thus, Qi can be considered a special neural response under certain conditions.

Commenting on practice, Chairman Mao said, "Things that are perceived cannot be immediately understood; only through understanding can deeper perception be achieved." Hence, further exploration into the sensation of Qi in Tai Chi Chuan is necessary. Whether Qi is bioelectricity or related to the meridians can be tested with meridian detection devices. The sensation of Qi, or "internal Qi," arises mainly because, during movements performed in a state of utmost relaxation, the stimulation of receptors around the blood vessels by nerve control, muscle contraction and relaxation, biochemical and bioelectrical changes increase blood vessel openness, sending excitation impulses to the brain's sensory centers, causing sensations of numbness, swelling, and warmth. Qi's circulation is closely related to vascular movement, aligning with traditional Chinese medicine concepts like "Where Qi goes, blood follows" and "Blood is the mother of Qi." If measured with a semiconductor thermometer, the extremities' temperature of someone experiencing Qi circulation during Tai

Chi practice can rise by half to one and a half degrees Celsius, evidencing the extensive opening of capillaries.

What are the benefits of Qi circulation? They include:

1. **Muscle capillary dynamics:** At rest, only about five out of thousands of capillaries per square millimeter of muscle have blood flowing through them, but this number can increase to two hundred during exercise. Capillaries open and close in a cyclical manner, functioning like millions of tiny hearts throughout the body. These "peripheral hearts" are as vital to life as the heart itself. Tai Chi Chuan's principle of "When one part moves, the whole body responds" helps reduce the heart's workload and lower blood pressure through extensive vascular opening.

2. **Enhanced focus and brain function:** Paying attention to Qi circulation during practice helps concentrate the mind, thereby regulating and strengthening brain neural activity.

3. **Improved metabolic processes** due to enhanced blood circulation, benefiting overall health and disease prevention.

To facilitate the circulation of Qi throughout the body, one must, during the practice of Tai Chi Chuan, concentrate the mind, relax the muscles, and execute movements slowly and evenly, guiding movements with intention. This aligns with what is stated in the "Inner Classic": "To relax the joints, soften the sinews, and harmonize the mind is to lead and guide the Qi." It echoes the ancient emphasis on calm and unhurried practice. By maintaining correct postures, it is not difficult to reach the state where "the bones are properly aligned, the sinews are soft, and the Qi and blood flow freely."

However, one should not overemphasize the role of Qi to an inappropriate extent, as the health benefits of Tai Chi Chuan are multifaceted. It should also be noted that other forms of exercise, though they may not involve the sensation of moving Qi, can offer the first and third benefits discussed above. Experience has shown that some individuals, after practicing Tai

Chi Chuan for an extended period and recovering from illness, do not report any sensation of Qi movement. Thus, the presence and clarity of Qi movement, besides the method of practice, are also related to an individual's constitution. In such cases, one might adopt the method of "balancing exercise" to swiftly experience a sensation of Qi and blood movement. The practice involves standing with feet parallel and slightly wider than shoulder-width apart, arms raised naturally to the sides, and the body relaxed. Then, slowly bend the body to the left and right, with the arms moving up and down like a seesaw (as illustrated in Illustration 10).

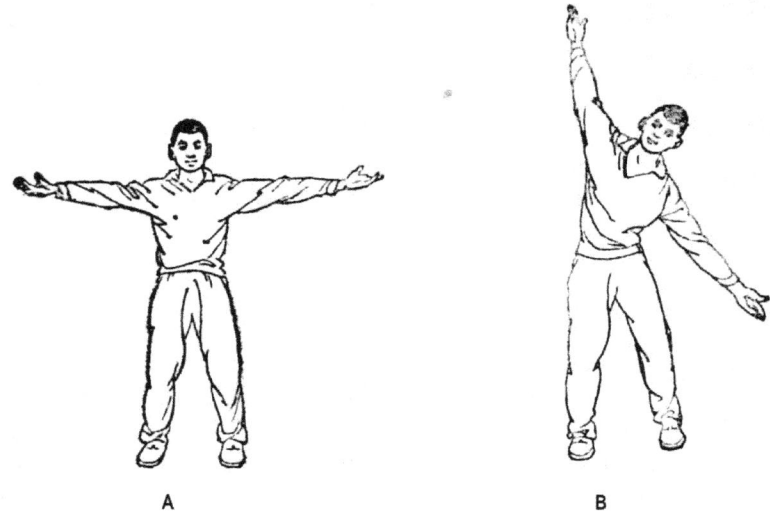

A                                    B

*Illustration 10*

After bending to one side, the arm on the bent side should feel warm and possibly turn redder, indicating congestion, while the color of the upper arm gradually becomes paler. Only then should the body slowly straighten. As the arms return to being raised to the sides, the paler arm may experience sensations similar to crawling insects or warmth, indicative of Qi and blood movement. To encourage the sensation of Qi and blood movement in the legs, adopting an empty stance and practicing with relaxed shoulders and elbows can help sink the Qi to the waist and abdomen. Relaxing the waist and hips, tucking in the buttocks, maintaining an upright torso, slightly bending the knees, and slightly turning them inward can help direct the Qi to the toes of the rear leg. If there is still no sensation of Qi and blood movement, do not force it; practicing with intention rather than exertion can also yield health and healing benefits.

## 24. What are the Benefits of Mind-led Movement in Tai Chi Chuan?

The essence of human consciousness is described as "the function of a particularly complex material known as the human brain." (Lenin, "Materialism and Empirio-criticism," Collected Works, Volume 2, p. 232). The physiological processes of brain activity are inseparable from the processes of consciousness; the former constitutes the material foundation of the latter, which in turn is the active product of the former.

Practicing Tai Chi Chuan with an emphasis on mental intent rather than brute force is simpler and less prone to the pitfalls of rigidity, making it crucial for widespread adoption. Tai Chi movements are conducted under the guidance of consciousness, or in other words, under the control of the brain. For instance, the seemingly simple movement of "Commencing Form" must be initiated by a gentle mental guidance: the arms are raised in front of the body, followed by squatting, bending the knees, and relaxing the waist. The elbows lead the hands in a gentle downward press, while the upper body remains upright. With proficiency, one can further synchronize this movement with exhalation and the downward movement of "Qi" to the area below the navel, as the legs gently grip the ground, simulating the sensation of "Qi" being drawn up to the lower abdomen. This is what is referred to as "Qi sinking to the Dantian." However, for beginners or those who do not yet perceive the circulation of Qi and blood, it suffices to focus on the leading role of the mind. This embodies the principle of "mind moves, body follows" and "each movement is mindful and intentional," as emphasized in traditional theory. Therefore, Tai Chi Chuan is not merely a physical exercise but places a greater emphasis on mental engagement, suggesting that the most crucial aspect of Tai Chi Chuan is to exercise the nervous system.

Besides motor and sensory functions, the nervous system also performs what is known as a nutritional function. The trophic nerves can influence the metabolism within the body, regulate the nutrition of tissues and organs, and are of significant importance to the body's capacity for activity. This function of the nervous system holds particular significance during physical exercise, as the heightened activity of the body necessitates enhanced nutrition to all organs and systems, increasing the chemical changes and metabolism between tissues and their environment. The significant therapeutic and fitness benefits of Tai Chi Chuan are closely linked to this integration of consciousness and movement. Such practice can stimulate a specific area of the cerebral cortex, inducing a protective inhibitory state in other regions of the brain. This not only allows the brain to rest but also helps eliminate pathological excitations caused by diseases in the cerebral cortex. It is important to note that mere rest and inhibition often fail to achieve optimal health benefits. Practice has shown that Tai Chi Chuan exercises are significantly more effective in certain cases than Pavlov's sleep therapy. Thus, stimulation of the central nervous system function and active training can help revive functions that have been suppressed or deteriorated by disease, thereby adjusting the functions of various systems and achieving therapeutic and fitness goals.

## 25. How can we achieve "Unity of Mind and Qi"?

It is crucial to emphasize that one should not overly concentrate on the flow of "Qi"; similarly, the guidance of consciousness in movement should not be excessively focused, as this may accelerate the onset of fatigue and lead to stiffness. The correct approach involves allowing "Qi" and consciousness to operate in the same manner as muscle movements—alternating between tension and relaxation, subtly guiding with intermittent presence and absence. For example, in the movement of "Brush Knee and Twist Step," consciousness should gradually intensify, focusing on the fingertips as the palm reaches its final position. At this moment, sensations such as tingling at the fingertips indicate the significant movement of "Qi." As the arm is withdrawn, consciousness should gradually fade, allowing for a momentary focus on the flow of "Qi" or simply letting go of the awareness of "Qi." This is what is referred to as the "unity of mind and Qi," implying that the interchange between the two should be lively and spirited to enjoy the full essence of movement, embodying the principle of alternating between the substantial and the insubstantial.

Harmonizing mind and Qi with movement not only provides a comprehensive exercise for both the internal and external aspects of the body but also enhances the interest in this activity. Prolonged practice of Tai Chi Chuan often leads to an engrossing passion that is hard to give up, which is one of the reasons Tai Chi Chuan is effective in treating some chronic illnesses.

However, for those who do not feel "Qi" or whose sensation of "Qi" is not clear during practice, achieving "unity of mind and Qi" is not a necessity. The concept of "unity of mind and Qi" or "leading Qi with the mind" is just one of the methods in the practice of Tai Chi Chuan and should not be pursued to the extent of causing stiffness. Individuals in this situation can practice Tai Chi Chuan with the method of "leading the body with the mind," which not only aids in achieving movements that are light and relaxed but can also yield favorable results (for more on "Qi," see sections 23 and 33 of this chapter).

## 26. How to Achieve "Rooted in the Feet, Generated in the Legs, Governed by the Waist, Manifested in the Fingers.

When practicing forms or push hands in Tai Chi Chuan, the source of strength originates from the feet. The feet grip the ground, generating a reactive force from the ground through the feet, legs, waist, and hands, thus producing power. Therefore, the saying "Rooted in the feet, generated in the legs, governed by the waist, manifested in the fingers" has a mechanical basis. This principle is easily understood in everyday life. For instance, a heavily loaded cart cannot be pushed with hands alone; force must be exerted through the feet, and only through the coordinated effort of the legs, waist, and hands can the cart be moved.

There are various opinions on how to meet this requirement in practice. Here, we provide the following perspectives for consideration:

For simplified Tai Chi Chuan, the 88 forms, Yang, Wu, and Sun styles, one should follow the steps discussed above and meet the requirements for the waist, back, shoulders, elbows, wrists, and hands. For Chen, Wu (Hao), Zhao Bao, and Jinling styles, a simpler method for the path of force involves: when stepping forward, the heel touches down first, the calf relaxes downward, then the foot gradually makes contact with the ground from the outer edge to the little toe, and so on until the big toe, each toe pressing down in turn. The Yongquan point (arch of the foot) lifts slightly as the toes grip the ground. This creates a dynamic where the toes and heel grip the ground firmly, while the arch lifts slightly, known as "solidity containing emptiness." When stepping back, the big toe touches down first, followed by the other toes and the outer edge to the heel in sequence, with the Yongquan point also lifting slightly. The path of force moves from the left foot and leg, through the waist to the right hand, and from the right foot and leg through the waist to the left hand. The waist acts as the central axis, similar to the fulcrum of scissors.

For those who find the action of gently gripping the ground with their toes too tense and uncomfortable, the practice of "relaxing the feet to allow the flow of Qi and blood" is recommended. This involves standing naturally with the feet flat on the ground, the toes relaxed without actively gripping the ground or lifting the Yongquan point, and the weight comfortably centered on the arch of the foot. As long as the body is upright and relaxed, this method of practice is also effective.

Regarding the practice of manifesting in the fingers, if the little finger leads, then the ring finger, middle finger, index finger, and finally the thumb follow in sequence; for movements drawing upwards and back, the thumb leads with a crushing motion, guiding the flow of force and blood from the thumb, index finger, middle finger, ring finger to the little finger, and finally through to the fingertips. The hook hand movement starts from the little finger to the ring finger, middle finger, index finger, and thumb, extending to the back of the wrist.

As the posture transitions and retracts, the Qi and blood also retract from the Yongquan point through the inside of the legs, perineum, to the area between the lower abdomen and waist. Here, the area between the lower abdomen and waist serves as the central hub, "the waist as the axle, the Qi and strength as the wheels," enabling the whole body to be interconnected by a single flow of Qi.

For those who perceive the flow of Qi and blood, following the described path of Qi and blood flow should not be difficult, even for practitioners of other Tai Chi Chuan styles. For those who do not feel the flow of Qi and blood, the method of "focus on the mind, not on the Qi" can be employed. That is, using intention to meticulously follow the outlined path, which can also achieve the effect of concentrated attention.

## 27. How many breathing methods are there in Tai Chi?

Tai Chi Chuan incorporates several approaches to breathing, each with its unique benefits and applications. Understanding these methods can enhance one's practice, aligning physical movements with internal energy flow for improved health and martial prowess.

### Natural Breathing Method

Breathing regulation is a complex process influenced by mental state, emotional stimuli, cardiovascular function, body fluids, hormones, and metabolic byproducts. Accumulation of carbon dioxide, decreased oxygen levels, and various byproducts from muscle activity can stimulate and affect the rate and depth of respiration. This adjustment is unconsciously completed through the central nervous system, particularly the cerebral cortex and respiratory center, without the need for conscious efforts to change this delicate gas exchange process through accelerated or forced deep breathing. Hence, the advocacy for natural breathing in Tai Chi Chuan practice is quite reasonable. This method requires focusing on the movements during practice, allowing breathing to occur naturally without any forced or artificial interference. However, this type of natural breathing differs from the breathing at rest or during intense physical activity. Its subtlety lies in the relaxed, slow, and coordinated body movements, which are lively yet solemn, achieving a serene concentration. In such a state of dynamic stillness and profound mental calm, breathing naturally deepens, akin to the natural deep breathing during sleep. Sleep breathing becomes naturally deep partly due to reduced metabolism (which differs from during Tai Chi practice) and partly because of the brain's relative tranquility.

This breathing method is broadly applicable and facilitates the popularization of Tai Chi Chuan. It is essential for beginners and also suitable for the elderly, those with physical weaknesses, or anyone practicing Tai Chi for health and healing purposes.

## Regulated Natural Deep Breathing Method

Regulated natural deep breathing involves intentionally deepening the breath gradually without disrupting its natural rhythm. This method should only be adopted after becoming proficient in the forms and can be synchronized with movements. However, it's crucial that the depth and synchronization with movements are not forced. Occasional shifts back to natural breathing can help prevent discomfort due to improper integration. This method is also broadly applicable for popularizing and advancing Tai Chi practice. When used by middle-aged and elderly practitioners, emphasis should be on shorter inhalations and longer, heavier exhalations. Extending exhalation helps expel more gases from the lungs, allowing for the intake of more air and improving pulmonary ventilation efficiency, thus preventing symptoms like chest tightness and rapid breathing. Additionally, it can enhance pulmonary elasticity and function during decline, offering some prevention against pulmonary emphysema. Given that lung capacity starts to decrease from the age of 35, proactive measures against age-related pulmonary emphysema are advised.

## Reverse Abdominal Breathing Method

Many advocate for the reverse abdominal breathing method during Tai Chi Chuan. This method is opposite to normal breathing, with the abdomen gradually retracting during a slow inhalation and protruding during exhalation, in contrast to the natural expansion during inhalation and contraction during exhalation of regular breathing. Some describe reverse breathing as the abdomen retracting and the diaphragm rising during inhalation, and the diaphragm descending during exhalation, inadvertently adding a chest breathing component. Further investigation and observation under X-ray revealed that, whether for regular or reverse breathing, the diaphragm descends during inhalation and ascends during exhalation, with exceptions in cases of diaphragmatic hernia, excessive abdominal pressure, or paralysis, which are rare in healthy individuals. Thus, the description of reverse abdominal breathing needs further exploration. The claim that reverse abdominal breathing increases the activity range of abdominal and diaphragmatic muscles, deepening the breath, also requires more observation. X-ray studies showed that the diaphragmatic movement in extreme reverse deep breathing was slightly less compared to regular deep breathing. Measurements of lung capacity in different deep breathing techniques indicated a slight increase in only one instance of reverse breathing, with most showing a decrease. This aligns with the understanding that a one-centimeter descent of the diaphragm increases chest volume by 250-300 milliliters, suggesting the observed decrease in lung capacity is consistent. While breathing during X-ray observation and lung capacity measurement may differ from that during Tai Chi practice, these findings prompt further investigation into the health benefits of reverse breathing. Preliminarily, if applied correctly, this method could strengthen diaphragmatic and abdominal muscles, increasing abdominal pressure variability, improving abdominal blood circulation, and facilitating the "Qi sinking to the lower abdomen" practice.

This reverse breathing method is suitable for those accustomed to it and may be particularly beneficial for individuals with gastroptosis.

In summary, while these three breathing methods share commonalities, each has its distinctive features. Their application should be tailored to individual physical conditions, health issues, and martial arts proficiency. Regardless of the chosen method, breathing should be comfortable, unforced, and progress gradually. Only through such an approach can one aid in health and healing and master the breathing methods of Tai Chi Chuan effectively.

## 28. Is the statement "breathing in and out of the mouth" correct?

In the nuanced practice of Tai Chi Chuan, the mastery of breath control is a cornerstone of both martial proficiency and holistic well-being. Addressing the question, "Is it correct to breathe through the mouth?", it is crucial to understand the intricacies of this subject from the perspective of a seasoned Tai Chi Chuan practitioner. The notion that breathing should be performed through the mouth carries a degree of oversimplification. Ordinarily, mouth breathing is seen as an unsanitary practice. Nevertheless, for Tai Chi enthusiasts dedicated to honing rapid, powerful strikes and delving into the martial aspects such as push hands, there are instances during intense physical exertion where breathing through the mouth, in tandem with the nose, becomes indispensable. For novices, whose familiarity with movements and breathing techniques is still developing, occasional reliance on mouth breathing to facilitate breath adjustment is permissible. However, this should be viewed as an adjunct rather than a substitute for nasal breathing. A hybrid approach to breathing is recommended, emphasizing inhalation through the nose and exhalation through the mouth with air gently escaping through slightly parted teeth. If medical conditions impede nasal breathing, seeking prompt treatment is advisable. In situations where mouth breathing becomes a necessity, the lips should be minimally opened, allowing air to flow softly through the openings in the teeth.

For practitioners pursuing Tai Chi Chuan for its therapeutic and fitness benefits, nasal breathing is advocated. This method ensures deep, sustained breaths. The secretions of the nasal mucosa add moisture to the inhaled air, while nasal hairs and mucosal secretions filter out dust, bacteria, and impurities, cleansing the air that enters the lungs. The nasal cavity's complex structure, enriched with a dense network of blood vessels, warms the air, aligning its temperature closer to that of the body. These nasal functions become especially critical during colder weather. Furthermore, mouth breathers often exhibit reduced diaphragmatic activity and poorly developed thoracic cages, underscoring the importance of rectifying this habit promptly.

## 29. Is the statement "movements and breathing must be integrated" correct?

The idea that movement and breathing must be integrated possesses a degree of one-sidedness. The coordination between movement and breathing should not be overly mechanical, ignoring the principles of adapting to the individual and flexible application. Furthermore, Tai Chi Chuan is not a form of breathing exercise but a martial art. The structure of a complete set of Tai Chi, including the arrangement of postures, continuity from one move to the next, and the integration of offensive and defensive intentions, is not solely devised based on coordinating with breathing. Hence, it's impractical to expect breathing to match every movement. Moreover, insisting on the integration of movement and breathing can hinder the widespread promotion and adoption of Tai Chi Chuan.

Should movements and breathing be integrated? Integration should occur naturally with certain movements where it is feasible. This approach allows movements to enhance respiratory function, while breathing, in turn, facilitates the transformation of movements to become more agile and grounded, also benefiting from the harmonious and invigorating effect of aligning mind, movement, and breath. However, for movements that do not naturally align with breathing, forcing them to match should be avoided to maintain the natural rhythm and harmony of both breathing and movement.

Different Tai Chi sequences vary in the frequency and depth of breathing; even within the same sequence, individuals of different physiques and levels of training should not be forced into uniformity. Generally, breathing naturally coordinates with movements that involve storing and releasing energy or are clearly defined in their execution. If practicing a sequence allows for a quarter to half of the movements to integrate with breathing, it is considered very good and can yield substantial health benefits. In reality, many long-term practitioners cannot achieve a close coordination of intent, movement, and breathing throughout an entire set. Forced mechanical integration would only lead to unnatural interference with breathing or result in disjointed movements, breaking the flow and coherence, especially in faster-paced Tai Chi styles.

For beginners, the focus should be on concentrating the mind and memorizing the movements without paying attention to breathing. Once the movements are memorized, the emphasis shifts to thinking and executing simultaneously, paying attention to the details and processes of each movement. This includes not just the changes in the fullness and emptiness of body movements but also integrating intent with movement. If the sequence is not yet fluent, forcing the integration of movement and breathing can lead to a loss of focus, increase mental strain, and make both posture and breathing harder to master, as tension can hinder and disrupt natural and deep breathing.

## 30. How should breathing coordinate with movements in Tai Chi Chuan?

In Tai Chi Chuan, the integration of breathing with movements naturally arises from the dynamics of the movements themselves. Often, those who do not initially focus on coordinating their breathing with movements will find themselves naturally aligning the two as they continue to practice. To facilitate mastery of this essential aspect, here are some general principles for coordinating breathing with movements:

## Inhalation during These Movements:

1. Rising movements,

2. Bending the arms,

3. Lifting the legs.

## Exhalation duringThese Movements:

1. Squatting movements,

2. Extending the arms (punching, pushing),

3. Stepping movements and when a movement reaches its final position.

In essence, inhale during posture transitions and exhale when pushing the palm or fist forward. Aim for inhalations to be light and short, and exhalations to be heavier and longer. In faster-paced Tai Chi practices, it's advisable to find a rhythm where several movements correspond to a single breath cycle, aligning both with physiological needs and martial principles. Tai Chi's distinctive feature is its smooth, agile, yet grounded movements. Breathing in a relaxed and gradual manner naturally fosters this agility, greatly benefiting posture transitions. Experienced practitioners can readily attest to this. For instance, during bathing or swimming, practicing inhalation and exhalation exercises can vividly demonstrate how the body lightens and floats with inhalation, and becomes heavier and sinks with exhalation. The body's specific gravity is similar to water, fluctuating between 0.96—0.99 during inhalation and 1.02—1.115 during exhalation. The same principle applies in the air, where breathing can induce sensations of lightness or heaviness. Lightening during inhalation aids in agility, whereas heaviness during exhalation contributes to stability and power generation. Additionally, studies have shown that muscular strength is greater during exhalation than inhalation. Understanding this underlines the logic behind principles such as "exhalation naturally leads to sinking," "flexibility follows breath control," and "strikes delivered during exhalation are more powerful."

The principle of inhaling with posture changes and exhaling with forward strikes should be adapted to individual circumstances. Young, healthy individuals or those who prefer faster movements might opt for the first method. For example, in the simplified Tai Chi move "Wild Horse Parts Mane," inhale while adopting a side-holding ball position, and exhale as the arms separate and strike forward. Elderly, physically weaker individuals, or those with chronic conditions, and those who favor slower movements can adopt the second method. Using "Wild Horse Parts Mane" as an example again, inhale at the start of the movement change and exhale upon completing the ball-holding position, with inhalation occurring as the hands prepare to separate and exhale upon completion of the step and final hand position.

For instance, in the 88-form Tai Chi Chuan, inhalation commonly occurs during rising movements, such as after completing "Needle at Sea Bottom" or "Step Forward and Plant Punch," and during arm retraction, whether one or both arms, as seen in movements like "Grasp the Sparrow's Tail" press and "Single Whip" left arm retraction. Exhalation is required during squatting actions and when extending one or both arms, indicating punches or palm strikes, such as in "Grasp the Sparrow's Tail" palm press, "Single Whip" left hand push, and punches in "Parry and Punch," "Punch Groin," and "Step Forward and Plant Punch."

These examples illustrate general tendencies, but actual coordination between each movement may vary, influenced by the pace and amplitude of movements, and individual lung capacity. Adaptation should be flexible based on specific circumstances.

When integrating breathing with movements, breathing should not be forced, held back, or strained. Although breathing is consciously regulated, it should naturally align with movements. If combining breathing and movements causes chest tightness or dizziness, do not force it. Instead, focus on relaxation and adopt a naturally calm and even breathing pattern, which, as mentioned, will naturally deepen with smooth and gentle movements. For individuals with severe pulmonary tuberculosis, movements should not be coordinated with breathing, relying entirely on natural breathing patterns.

## 31. How do you Understand 'Opening with Inhalation, Closing with Exhalation' versus 'Closing with Inhalation, Opening with Exhalation'

How to harmonize breathing with movement remains a topic of diverse opinions. Some practitioners advocate for 'Opening with Inhalation, Closing with Exhalation,' while others support the reverse—'Closing with Inhalation, Opening with Exhalation.' Each camp holds steadfast to its views, leading to a conundrum for learners.

Those who support 'Closing with Inhalation, Opening with Exhalation' believe that movements involving bending, retreating, storing energy, rising, transforming, and drawing in correspond with 'closing' and should be paired with inhalation. Conversely, extending, advancing, descending, dropping, releasing, and solidifying movements correspond with 'opening' and should be paired with exhalation. For instance, in the Simplified Tai Chi Chuan, one inhales as the hands part and draw back in a movement akin to sealing, and exhales as the hands push forward. This aligns with the common martial theory that inhalation is associated with closing and storing, whereas exhalation is associated with opening and releasing.

On the other hand, proponents of 'Opening with Inhalation, Closing with Exhalation' argue that the combination of breath and movement should be guided by the expansion and contraction of the chest cavity. Movements that expand the chest are considered 'opening' and should be paired with inhalation; movements that contract the chest are seen as 'closing' and should be paired with exhalation. For example, in Sun Style Tai

Chi Chuan, inhalation accompanies opening movements, and exhalation accompanies closing movements. 'Opening' movements expand the chest, while 'closing' movements contract it. In martial application, 'opening' is associated with drawing in, transforming, and storing, whereas 'closing' is associated with advancing, solidifying, and releasing. This is encapsulated in the phrase, 'On drawing in, position oneself to be empty; on closing, release immediately.'

In summary, though the two viewpoints on the synchronization of movement and breath seem contradictory, their practical applications largely agree. Both emphasize inhaling during drawing in, transforming, and storing movements, and exhaling during releasing and solidifying movements. The primary difference lies in their interpretations of 'opening' and 'closing.' Essentially, 'opening' and 'closing' are just expansions and contractions, respectively. Traditionally, 'opening' is an outward expansion, while 'closing' is an inward contraction—expanding is opening, and contracting is closing. It must be acknowledged that the simplistic concept of opening and closing has been overly complicated in the past, especially when intertwined with breathing, leading to confusion. As highlighted earlier, the opening and closing of the arms do not always align with the expansion and contraction of the chest cavity, hence there's no need to be entangled in the debate between 'Opening with Inhalation, Closing with Exhalation' and 'Closing with Inhalation, Opening with Exhalation.'

## 32. What Are the Benefits of Natural Deep Breathing in Tai Chi Chuan?

In practicing Tai Chi Chuan, regardless of the breathing method employed, one can cultivate natural and deep breathing, which holds significant value in health preservation and disease treatment. Firstly, these breathing techniques not only strengthen the respiratory organs but, more importantly, they enhance the cardiovascular system, ensuring that it is not overburdened by physical activity.

Breathing evenly, quietly, deeply, and lengthily during practice stimulates the diaphragm and the movements of the chest and abdomen, increasing the capacity for gas exchange in the lungs. Studies have shown that elderly individuals who regularly practice Tai Chi Chuan exhibit greater chest breathing capacity and lung volume compared to their peers, experience lighter breathlessness during standardized activities, and recover more quickly. This indicates that regular practice strengthens the chest respiratory muscles and the diaphragm, improves lung tissue elasticity, lowers the rate of rib cartilage ossification, and enhances thoracic mobility, all of which are of great significance in preventing emphysema.

The intensified movement of the diaphragm and chest abdomen also accelerates the return flow of venous blood, improving the blood circulation of the heart itself. Tai Chi Chuan has been proven to have a therapeutic effect on certain heart diseases, a fact supported not only by practice but also by cardiovascular function tests and electrocardiograms. Additionally, the increased movement range of the diaphragm enhances the blood flow to the organs in the abdominal cavity, such as the stomach, liver, and spleen, improving their absorption functions. Many individuals suffering from gastrointestinal dyspepsia or chronic enteritis have been completely cured through long-term practice of Tai Chi Chuan, serving as a compelling testament to its benefits.

Natural deep breathing, aside from facilitating metabolism and timely oxygen replenishment, also effectively calms and strengthens the nervous system. It plays an active role in eliminating fatigue and preventing and treating hypertension. Studies have shown that elderly individuals who regularly practice Tai Chi Chuan have lower average blood pressure and a reduced rate of arteriosclerosis.

## 33. What is "Qi sinking in Dantian" and How Is It Practiced and Understood?

In the past, many people in the martial arts and medical fields advocated "Qi sinks to the Dantian," but the position of the Dantian was not consistently agreed upon. For example, "Shimen is the Dantian, also called Mingmen, located two inches below the navel" (Li Binhui's "Study of the Eight Extraordinary Meridians"); "Three inches below the navel is called Dantian" ("Essentials of Life and Nature"); "One inch three fen is the Dantian" ("Huangting Sutra"); "Above the seven sections is the small heart, below the Shenque is the Dantian" ("Dan Sutra"); "Dantian is in front of the kidneys and behind the navel" ("Red Furnace Point Snow"); in addition, there are also "the intersection of the Chong and Dai meridians is the Dantian," and so on.

The term "Dantian" contains the idealistic color of Taoist alchemy and immortality. In ancient times, when people practiced to a certain extent, they often felt warmth and other special sensations in the lower abdomen. At that time, without a scientific explanation, they placed their fantasy of immortality on this slight sensation and compared it to the so-called elixir of immortality refined in a furnace, beautifully named "internal elixir." Thus, they called this so-called place of refining the internal elixir "Dantian." Of course, this name is unscientific; there is no such thing as an elixir of immortality or internal elixir in the world. However, we should strip away its superstitious coat and adopt its health-beneficial exercise methods.

As for the different experiences of each person, besides individual differences, it is mainly because the sensory nerves in the abdomen are visceral nerves, one characteristic of which is that the reflections transmitted to the brain's sensory center are not so accurate and often have errors. For example, in the early stages of appendicitis, some patients feel pain in the stomach or navel, which is different from the actual anatomical position of the appendix. Therefore, the exploration and debate on the exact position of the Dantian are unnecessary, and the different records of the Dantian's position are understandable.

What does the "Qi" in "Qi sinks to the Dantian" refer to? It is definitely not the air we breathe because the air we breathe cannot reach the abdominal cavity. The "Qi" in "Qi sinks to the Dantian" is just a kind of nerve reflection in the lower abdomen when practicing martial arts. Therefore, changing "Qi sinks to the Dantian" to "Qi sinks to the lower abdomen" is more appropriate. Why is there this reflection in the lower abdomen? Let me explain as follows.

Some people experience Qi sinking to the lower abdomen when inhaling. Due to practicing martial arts, the breathing gradually becomes naturally deep and long, and the diaphragm descends more during inhalation, which gives the internal organs in the abdomen a beneficial gentle squeezing and massage effect. This squeezing and massage can also stimulate the receptors in the abdominal cavity, turning into bioelectric pulses, transmitted to the brain's sensory center through sensory fibers, thus causing the sensation of Qi rushing to the lower abdomen, which is the so-called "Qi sinks to the Dantian" (see page 49). Therefore, some people think that "Qi sinks to the Dantian" is a kind of deep breathing exercise. When inhaling, coordinating with adjusting the crotch, gently lifting the perineum with intention, and relaxing when exhaling, making the perineum lift and relax in coordination with breathing, will have greater benefits, and has some effects on the prevention and treatment of longevity and certain chronic reproductive system diseases.

It is relatively easy to grasp Qi sinking to the lower abdomen when exhaling. Due to the diaphragm rising during exhalation, the anal muscles relaxing, the abdominal pressure decreasing, and the closed capillaries in the abdominal cavity suddenly opening, it causes a warm nerve sensation in the abdomen, which is the so-called "Qi sinks to the lower abdomen." In addition, exhaling has a counterforce on the lungs, similar to the recoil force formed on the cannon body when a shell is fired, which may also be the source of the "diaphragm naturally descending during exhalation" sensation. This counterforce, combined with the postures of sinking shoulders and elbows, containing the chest and pulling the back, and keeping the tailbone upright, especially the ribs naturally sinking forward and downward in an arc with the exhalation movement, gathering towards the lower abdomen, all help form the sensation of "Qi sinks to the lower abdomen" during exhalation.

However, "Qi sinks to the lower abdomen" should not be rushed. It must not be done as "Qi penetrates the Dantian" or "forcefully enters the Dantian." Sinking and penetrating are different; sinking comes from nature, penetrating comes from force. Sinking is like something descending in still water due to gravity, while "forcefully entering" will further disrupt natural breathing. Below are two methods to help grasp "Qi sinks to the lower abdomen."

1. The practice method of "Qi sinks to the lower abdomen" when inhaling—stand with feet shoulder-width apart, slightly bend the knees, hands can overlap and gently touch the lower abdomen, or can respectively touch the sides of the navel in a slight ball-holding posture, using intention to gently guide the lower abdomen's rise and fall movement with breathing. This way, through the external sensory receptors of the abdominal wall skin, it gives the brain a specific local impulse sensation, closely linking the lower abdomen with the brain, and the conditioned reflex of abdominal breathing will form more quickly, making it easier to practice the above method of "Qi sinks to the lower abdomen" when inhaling.

2. The practice method of "Qi sinks to the lower abdomen" when exhaling—stand with feet shoulder-width apart, palms facing up and gently lifting when inhaling, arms continuing to move when starting to exhale, turning the palms and gently bending to hug in front of the chest, fingers touching the chest wall, then slowly squatting down with the exhalation, while gradually and gently pressing the hands to the lower abdomen; repeating this practice will help quickly grasp "Qi sinks to the lower abdomen" when exhaling.

Whether it is "Qi sinks to the lower abdomen" when inhaling or exhaling, if mastered correctly, it will have certain health benefits just like the operation of Qi. Because it increases the movement of the diaphragm, it can not only enhance the ventilation function of the lungs but also benefit the blood circulation of the internal organs in the chest and abdomen due to the rhythmic changes in abdominal pressure, especially for the elderly with rib cartilage ossification and thoracic activity disorders and patients with emphysema.

Due to the increased range of diaphragm movement, the internal organs naturally descend slightly during inhalation, lowering the body's center of gravity, and due to the counterforce of the exhalation airflow on the lungs and the ribs naturally sinking forward and downward in an arc, it can achieve a similar stable balance effect like a roly-poly toy. Therefore, "intention in the lower abdomen" during turning can also help maintain body balance.

It must be pointed out that practicing Tai Chi is not about sinking Qi downward from beginning to end, but as the movement progresses and breathing changes, sometimes Qi sinks downward, sometimes Qi rises upward, all forming naturally and unintentionally, making it easier for the body to rise and fall and switch between emptiness and solidity. Through long-term practice, it can improve the flexibility of movements and achieve fitness effects. How can one make the intention and Qi sometimes reach the limbs and sometimes inject into the lower abdomen and waist during specific practice? Take the method of "Qi sinks to the lower abdomen" when inhaling as an example: when extending the hand outward, the intention guides the arm outward, if someone has a sense of Qi, at this time, Qi and intention will reach the fingertips, while coordinating with exhalation; when retracting the hand inward, the intention slowly guides the hand inward, and by the way, shifts the intention to the abdomen (the diaphragm descending during inhalation can also play some auxiliary role), if someone has a sense of Qi, at this time, there will be a sense of "Qi sinks to the lower abdomen." Those without a sense of Qi can use the method of "intention sinks to the lower abdomen," which can also achieve the effect of internal mental focus. In addition, some people do not pay attention to the coordination of breathing and movements, only maintaining a relaxed and natural state of the chest and abdomen at all times, which can also achieve good fitness effects.

## 34. How Does Tai Chi Chuan Benefit the Skin?

The skin not only protects internal tissues and regulates body temperature through sweating, but it is also covered with sensory nerve endings that receive pain, temperature, and touch sensations, making it one of our body's sensory organs. The skin as a sensory organ, especially as a touch organ, like other sensory organs, is an intermediary between the external environment and our perception, allowing us to form concepts about stimuli from external objects. The large number of different types of receptors in the skin are closely connected to the brain, spinal cord, and autonomic nervous system. For example, when we accidentally touch a hot object with our arm, the receptors in the arm's skin quickly transmit the stimulus along the afferent nerves to the spinal cord, allowing us to reflexively withdraw our arm without careful analysis.

The skin can not only trigger defensive reflexes, but any changes in external conditions (such as cold, warmth, movement, mutual touching during push hands, etc.) can excite skin receptors, quickly changing the functional state of the central nervous system, producing various reactions, and readjusting the tissues of the body's internal organs.

Healthy skin plays a significant role in the overall state of the body, and the various functions performed by the skin are related to the condition of the entire organism.

In martial arts, there are sayings like "internally cultivate one breath, externally train sinews, bones, and skin" or "internally cultivate one breath, externally train one layer of skin," which fully embodies the importance martial arts places on training respiratory organs and sinews and bones, as well as the various functions of the skin. The push hands practice in Tai Chi is both an active exercise and a mutually comfortable passive massage, therefore it has a good effect on training the functions of skin receptors and can enhance their sensitive responses. When practicing the form, due to the focus on relaxation and mental calmness and concentration, some people can experience the air resistance against their palm movements when practicing in a quiet environment. This type of practice also has some effect on further concentrating thoughts and stabilizing the mind.

## 35. How to Understand 'Everywhere There Is Emptiness and Fullness'?

What does 'emptiness' mean? Emptiness refers to being flexible and soft. And what about 'fullness'? Fullness implies being tense and firm. In a certain sense, emptiness is to be relaxed, and fullness is to be tense.

In the movement of Tai Chi Chuan, emptiness and fullness are complementary, interdependent, and form a contradictory unity. During motion, a certain group of muscles contracts while another group relaxes simultaneously; without this opposition, movement cannot be completed. Therefore, in Tai Chi Chuan, whether it be the upper limbs, lower limbs, trunk, or any part of the body, emptiness and fullness exist everywhere — this is the essence of 'everywhere there is emptiness and fullness.'

Taking the lower limbs as an example, if the left leg bears the body's weight or the majority of it, then the left leg is 'full,' and the right leg is 'empty'; if the body's weight shifts to the right leg, then the right leg becomes 'full,' and the left leg becomes 'empty.' For instance, in the 'Single Whip' stance, the left leg primarily bears the weight, making it 'full' and the right leg 'empty.' The same applies to the hands: if the focus is on the right hand, it becomes 'full,' and the left hand 'empty'; if the focus shifts to the left hand, then the left hand is 'full,' and the right hand 'empty.' Again, taking 'Single Whip' as an example, the left hand is 'full' and the right hand 'empty' because the focus is on the left hand. This is the initial step in distinguishing between emptiness and fullness. Even within the entire left hand, distinctions between emptiness and fullness are made, with the outer side of the left palm being 'full.' Thus, in the entire 'Single Whip' movement, there is a differentiation of emptiness and fullness between the left and right hands and legs, with further distinctions within the left hand itself, illustrating 'everywhere there is emptiness and fullness.'

The existence of emptiness and fullness in various parts of the body is not fixed in location and is transient in time, changing with the postures of Tai Chi Chuan. To achieve fluid changes between emptiness and fullness, one must further embrace 'emptiness within fullness and fullness within emptiness,' meaning there should be a conscious effort to maintain slight elasticity in muscle relaxation and tension for ease of joint and muscle transition. Concepts such as "the force seems relaxed but not relaxed, about to extend but not yet extended," "emptiness is not completely powerless, and fullness is not completely rigid," encapsulate this idea. When applying force in 'fullness,' it's important to measure and ensure it is not sluggish or stiff. Taking 'Single Whip' as an example, the left hand being 'full' means concentration is primarily on the left hand, and all parts that should not exert force must relax. The right hand being 'empty' must still be focused, maintaining warding off energy without loss. This 'emptiness within fullness' serves to balance the center of gravity and enhance the left hand's force application.

From a physiological perspective, if muscles remain tense and contracted for an extended period, it can impede biochemical processes and lead to rapid fatigue. Likewise, prolonged nervous system excitation without rest can induce protective inhibition, reducing muscle work capacity. Thus, muscles should work in coordination during movements, with tension and relaxation alternating, meaning emptiness and fullness must change constantly. This not only trains the central nervous system and bodily functions but also, through rhythmic cyclical work where muscle tension and relaxation alternate, helps restore muscle work capacity, providing a unique form of 'rest.' This benefits blood circulation: when muscles relax, blood flows easily into them, and when muscles tense, blood is actively transported back to the heart via veins.

In transitioning between emptiness and fullness, it's especially important to relax muscles not involved in the work timely, which plays a significant role in improving technique and offers many benefits. Relaxing muscles when not working reduces the physiological burden on the body. If antagonistic muscles actively relax when tensing, the braking effect on movement is minimized, saving the active force of muscles undertaking work. Additionally, relaxing antagonistic muscles increases joint flexibility, benefiting joint flexibility development.

Tai Chi Chuan demands high coordination. Only when muscles are free from excess tension can movements be performed smoothly and coherently. If muscle involvement is untimely or antagonistic muscles relax late, movements become constrained and rigid, affecting both muscle work capacity and movement accuracy.

In Push Hands, relying on focused concentration, transitions between emptiness and fullness become skillful. Emptiness and fullness manifest as defense and attack or emptiness and solidity, respectively. 'Emptiness' here means using 'emptiness' to meet the opponent's 'fullness,' causing their force to miss, encapsulated by 'if the left is heavy, then the left is empty; if the right is heavy, then the right is solid.' In Push Hands, one must not only embody 'emptiness within fullness and fullness within emptiness' within oneself but also grasp the opponent's state of emptiness and fullness, achieving targeted action.

In summary, to effectively apply the principles of emptiness and fullness within Tai Chi Chuan's Push Hands and each posture, one needs to practice over time to achieve a good grasp and application. The following points are offered for consideration:

1. Distinguish between the emptiness and fullness of the lower limbs in every movement. Regularly shifting the body weight onto one leg is also a good method to gradually strengthen the lower limbs.

2. Steps should not be too long or wide. If the distance between the two feet is too great, it becomes difficult to change steps and alternate between emptiness and fullness fluidly.

3. Maintain a centered and upright posture without leaning; learn to use intent rather than force, ensuring one foot is firmly planted before stepping with the other.

4. When physical strength and time permit, practice Push Hands more. This allows for a careful further experience of the changes and effects of emptiness and fullness in movement.

## 36. What is Double-Weighting? How Can It Be Avoided?

There is no consistent understanding of "double-weighted" in the Tai Chi community. Some believe that "double-weighted means when both hands use force in the same direction, or both feet use force in the same direction, it is called double-weighted. When only the hands use force in the same direction, it is double-weighted in the hands. When only the feet use force in the same direction, it is double-weighted in the feet. When both hands and feet use force in the same direction simultaneously, it is double-weighted in the whole body." This view is one-sided. According to this explanation, the "Starting Posture" in simplified Tai Chi would suffer from whole-body double-weightedness - wouldn't that mean the very first move is wrong?! Clearly this explanation is incorrect. The error lies in not distinguishing between "double sinking" and "double-weighted", mistakenly interpreting "double sinking" as "double-weighted".

The classics say "double-weighted leads to stagnation", but the "Starting Posture" has no feeling of stagnation, so how can it be called "double-weighted"? The "Explanation of Lightness, Heaviness, Floating and Sinking in Tai Chi" clearly states: "Double-weighted is a flaw, failing by being overly solid, different from sinking. Double sinking is not a flaw, aiming for emptiness, different from heaviness." This clearly distinguishes between "sinking" and "heaviness". "Overly solid" means "completely solid", "absolutely solid" or "pathologically solid", describing a solidness that has lost elasticity, belonging to an inflexible, unyielding force that does not meet Tai Chi requirements. Specifically, the horse stance in Tai Chi, the double pushing hands in Yang style Tai Chi's "Grasp Sparrow's Tail", the 88th form, and the double forward push in Wu, Yang and Sun style Tai Chi's "Apparent Closing" should all be called double sinking when done correctly (without losing elastic force), not "double-weighted". Only when the movements become stiff, heavy and inflexible can they be called "double-weighted". For example, if in the "horse stance" the feet are too far apart, sinking too much, losing the springy elastic force and affecting the flexibility of movement, it should be called "double-weighted". Even in the bow stance, if the feet are too far apart front to back, the bent knee goes past the toes losing elasticity and becoming stagnant, it does not meet Tai Chi requirements and suffers from the problem of "half-heavy and biased, stagnant and incorrect". In push hands, when butting heads occurs or steps are too large, losing flexible elasticity and becoming stagnant, it can also be called "double-weighted".

In short, anything that hinders the alternation of muscle tension and relaxation, causes movements to lose flexibility and coordination, or force to lose elastic peng energy, should be avoided. The "Tai Chi Classics" state: "To avoid this flaw (double-weightedness), one must understand yin and yang". This essentially refers to the need in practicing forms or push hands to allow the extensor and flexor muscle groups to fully function, complementing and opposing each other, facilitating the mutual transformation between contraction and relaxation of the two muscle groups. When this transformation is applied skillfully, it is the so-called "mutual support of yin and yang", reaching the state of "understanding force".

## 37. How to Understand and Achieve 'Coordination Between Upper and Lower Body, Whole-Body Harmony'?

In practicing Tai Chi Chuan, all movements must coordinate the upper limbs, lower limbs, and trunk, among other parts. This coordination is what is meant by the harmony between upper and lower body parts. This concept should not be narrowly interpreted as merely pertaining to the hands and feet. For example, in the 'Cloud Hands' movement, the hands move in a coordinated manner above and below each other. Beyond just the coordination of the upper and lower limbs, the hands themselves must follow this principle. Without the twisting of the waist, it would be impossible to execute the lifting, wrapping, turning, and pressing techniques in 'Cloud Hands.' Thus, coordination between upper and lower parts is a key principle in all Tai Chi movements, not just concerning the hands and feet, although their coordination is a significant aspect of whole-body harmony. Therefore, the principle of 'upper and lower body coordination and whole-body harmony' highlights a focal point while also being comprehensive.

In Tai Chi Chuan, the feet are like the roots of a plant, providing stability to the body. However, this stability is influenced by the coordination of all body parts and originates from the legs, infusing down to the feet. The waist serves as the central hub of the body, with energy generated by the waist traveling down through the legs to the feet and up through the shoulders and arms to the fingertips. Thus, in any movement, the whole body should act as one, expressing the reactive force from the ground as a unified energy, achieving the harmony between upper and lower parts and whole-body coordination.

What is the significance of this coordination?

Achieving harmony between upper and lower parts allows for advantageous positioning and coordinated movements, preventing the body technique from becoming disorganized. This can be analyzed from two perspectives:

1. **From a movement perspective**, Tai Chi Chuan is an exercise that provides a comprehensive workout for the body, not focusing on individual parts. Thus, achieving a full-body workout requires coordinated activity of the trunk and limbs. Every movement is an integrated activity, closely coordinating internal and external, upper and lower parts, allowing for balanced development of the body.

2. **In Push Hands,** only by achieving coordination between upper and lower parts can one seize the opportunity and gain an advantageous position. In other words, only when the body technique is unified, and advancing and retreating are appropriate, can Push Hands be successfully executed. The phrase "it is difficult for the opponent to advance when upper and lower parts move in harmony" emphasizes the importance of this coordination in offense and defense. If the body technique is disorganized and the hands and feet cannot cooperate, vulnerabilities will emerge, making it easy to be controlled by the opponent.

To achieve this coordination, consider the following points:

1. **Beginners should start with practicing individual forms** (such as the starting posture, warding off, Cloud Hands, etc.) to achieve coordination between the trunk and limbs. Additionally, practicing step work or stance training (such as standing in an empty stance, bow stance, etc.) is advisable to strengthen the lower limbs' support. Then, through continuous practice of all movements, coordinate the advancing and retreating step work with the rotation of the spine and waist. In any movement, ensure that the actions of the hands and feet are synchronized without precedence. A common mistake is moving the feet too quickly before the hands, resulting in slow hand movements or vice versa. Other errors include failing to move the bending of the knees and lowering of the waist in unison with the body. How can these issues be corrected? Mistakes often occur in the waist and legs, so constantly paying attention to the correct posture of the waist and legs can gradually lead to whole-body coordination. In movements where the center of gravity shifts forward, like in a bow stance, the extending of the back leg and the supporting of the front leg, elongating the waist before relaxing it, and the abdomen, chest, shoulders, and hands should move forward uniformly; when shifting the center of gravity backward, slightly withdraw the hip joint (femoral head), lower the waist and bend the knees, with the abdomen, chest, and shoulders moving back simultaneously. In turning movements, use the waist as the axis to drive the limbs, guiding the direction and energy of the movement. Beginners should especially ensure maintaining a certain lateral distance between the feet and an appropriate front-to-back distance, which is crucial for achieving upper and lower body coordination and flexible, stable rotation."

2. **Push Hands practice offers further opportunities to practice and experience the coordination between upper and lower body parts.** For instance, during two-person moving step

Push Hands, the techniques of the hands and the movements of the steps must be in sync. Advancing involves pressing, while retreating involves rolling back. There should be no delay whatsoever; otherwise, it becomes easy to be controlled by the opponent.

## 38. How to understand and achieve "internal and external harmony"?

'Internal' refers to the body's internal organs, especially the brain and its functions—spirit, psychology, consciousness. It must be emphasized that matter is primary, while spirit, psychology, and consciousness are secondary. Modern advanced neurophysiology has thoroughly debunked the idealistic notion that spirit, thought, and consciousness can exist independently of material conditions. Human thought and consciousness are characteristics of a highly organized material, the brain, and are products of brain activity developed on the basis of human social and historical practice and labor. They represent objective reality as reflected in the human brain. The reactivity of consciousness should also be noted. Once human consciousness arises in the labor process, it possesses an initiative that is manifested in various human activities.

Spirit depends on matter. Diseases in the brain or other organs undoubtedly affect the spirit. However, dialectical materialism acknowledges and values the reaction of the spirit, which in turn affects matter, influencing the brain's particularly complex matter and its functional state. Thus, it affects the regulation of other organs, influencing the respiratory system, cardiovascular system, endocrine system, metabolism, and a series of other physiological functions within the body.

In physical activity, the influence of spirit is more apparent. For example, take the simple activity of walking. Walking twenty miles in the same amount of time should theoretically cause the same amount of fatigue for the same person. However, the fatigue experienced while walking in a joyful state with friends compared to rushing to an appointment under stress, despite the same speed and distance, is vastly different. It's also observable in daily life that the same task can feel more exhausting when done in anger or frustration, and less so, or not at all, when done with joy.

Therefore, maintaining a spirit of revolutionary optimism and struggle is crucial in practicing Tai Chi Chuan, avoiding impatience and worry. Always maintain composure, tranquility, and joyfulness in practice, moving with stillness, concentrated yet relaxed. This calm and collected spirit is an effective remedy against the anxiety and pain caused by illness.

'External' broadly refers to the body's limbs and even includes the skin's surface.

Whether it's the body's whole or partial activity, even the slightest movement must be completed under the control of the nervous system. The method by which mental and physical movements are closely integrated under the unified command of the nervous system is 'Integration of Internal and External.' In a state of utmost mental comfort, movement is as smooth as flowing clouds and water, gentle and firm, lively yet refined, effortless, and enjoyable. Engaging in such activity daily will undoubtedly have therapeutic effects, improve work efficiency, extend working hours, and contribute more to the socialist revolution and construction.

## 39. How do we understand the phrase: "Where there is up, there is down; where there is front, there is back; where there is left, there is right"?

The phrase "where there is up, there is down; where there is front, there is back; where there is left, there is right" aligns with dialectics. Without down, there is no up; without back, there is no front; without right, there is no left, and vice versa. This principle is accurate in both stance training and Push Hands in Tai Chi. For instance, if there is "lightness and agility at the top," then there must be relaxation and sinking in the hips below, creating a sense of elongation between upper and lower parts. This facilitates the loosening of spinal joints, thereby benefiting posture changes during movement. Similarly, when the right hand is embracing upward and the left hand is pressing downward, the left hand should contain the springy force of pressing down, regardless of whether it makes contact with the opponent. This generates much greater force than using the warding-off energy of the right hand alone, exemplifying "where there is left, there is right." If the shifting energy in the arms is accompanied by the coordinated strength of the upper body and legs, it embodies "where there is up, there is down." When the left hand strikes forward, it is often effective for the right hand to pull back, lending power to the left-hand strike and integrating the rotational force of the waist and spine, which is "where there is front, there is back." However, it's essential to emphasize that amidst the various contradictions between up and down, front and back, left and right, it is necessary to identify the "principal contradiction and its principal aspect" based on the specific circumstances during Push Hands or form practice. Attention must be paid to the distinctiveness of movements, mastering the correct technique. For example, when the left hand strikes forward while the right hand retreats simultaneously, front and back transform into up and down. Among the contradictions of up and down, front and back, left and right, the main contradiction in the context of striking forward and pulling back often centers on the striking hand as the principal aspect of the contradiction, and so on.

## 40. How to Understand and Achieve 'Continuity without Interruption'?

'Continuity without Interruption' refers to the principle in Tai Chi Chuan that each movement and intention, as well as the application of energy, must be continuous (sometimes the energy ceases, but the intention does not).

From the beginning to the end of a Tai Chi Chuan form, each movement connects to the next without pause, aiming to be executed as one seamless flow. This continuous practice can only be achieved with focused concentration, thus it serves as an effective exercise for brain function.

Classical Tai Chi texts describe this unbroken continuity with phrases like "moving energy as if drawing silk," "from beginning to end, uninterrupted," "like the great Yangtze River, flowing endlessly," or "like drifting clouds and flowing water." However, like maintaining a uniform speed, continuity also exists relatively to other movements, especially in Chen-style Tai Chi Chuan. A posture often ends with a brief moment that seems to pause but doesn't truly stop, channeling intention to the fingertips, embodying 'the posture ends, but the intention continues,' or 'energy ends, but intention does not.' Without these brief pauses, movements can become hasty and superficial, making it difficult to achieve solidity and accuracy when issuing power. Therefore, some practitioners specifically advocate for a 'non-flowing water' approach to practice, referring to these brief pauses at the end of a posture. During form practice, although there's a brief pause upon completing a posture, the intention does not halt, avoiding the drawback of having to restart entirely. In the 88-form, as well as in Sun, Wu, Yang, and Wu (Hao) styles of Tai Chi Chuan, these pauses are not very pronounced, with some practitioners only slightly reducing speed at the completion of a posture to ensure the intention extends to the fingertips. In Push Hands, the continuous application of intention and movement leaves little opportunity for the opponent to attack, providing tight defense; on the other hand, it allows one to seek opportunities to counterattack at any moment.

How to achieve 'Continuity without Interruption'? The following methods are suggested for reference:

1. **Regular practice should be conducted without breaks.** All joints throughout the body should gradually loosen, smoothly transitioning from one to the next, creating a connected line. Any joint that does not move smoothly should be promptly corrected.

2. **Each posture can end with a very brief moment that seems to pause but doesn't truly stop.** However, the 'intention' must not be interrupted, meaning one's focus must remain constant without wandering even for an instant."

# 41. How to Master the pace in Tai Chi?

Many Tai Chi enthusiasts, both past and present, advocate practicing forms slowly. This may be because slowness makes it easier to achieve mental calmness, use intention rather than force, and relax both internally and externally, allowing one to gradually experience and correct areas of tension throughout the body. Consider that each movement requires relaxation in the skin, joints, and even internal organs and nervous system - achieving this level of relaxation without a certain slowness would be difficult and likely result in a lack of rootedness. Practicing Tai Chi with relaxation and tranquility can enhance sensory sensitivity and develop elastic, resilient explosive power. Only through slow movements can one carefully examine whether every part of the body is relaxed to the greatest extent possible, creating good conditions for tension (force generation) at any time, allowing one to quickly and flexibly concentrate force at a single point, thereby developing both strength and speed. From this perspective, slowness can be seen as nurturing quickness. Observations have shown that long-term Tai Chi practitioners have faster reaction times. The testing method used was: Tai Chi practitioners pressed a button as soon as they saw a light appear in front of them. This demonstrates that faster nerve conduction leads to quicker reactions and button pressing. Tai Chi practitioners' average reaction time was 333.2 milliseconds, while non-exercisers averaged over 400.0 milliseconds.

Mental calmness is key to achieving "quick response to quick movements, slow following of slow movements" in Tai Chi. However, this doesn't mean slowness can overcome speed. In push hands, quickness still generally prevails, but Tai Chi practitioners, through long-term practice of slow forms and push hands, achieve an understanding of energy and fully utilize the waist and spine as an axis with spiral force in advancing and retreating, making it difficult for opponents to perceive changes in force. This allows practitioners to easily maintain the initiative (or transform a passive situation into an active one), which is why even 70-80 year old practitioners can succeed in push hands.

Slowness also allows for naturally deep breathing, makes it easier to sink qi to the lower abdomen, and is a method for increasing or decreasing exercise intensity. Practicing with a low stance requires greater leg strength to support the body, and when combined with slow movements, the large leg muscle groups require even more forceful contraction and relaxation, resulting in a high-intensity workout. Even some long-time soccer players or long fist practitioners initially find their leg strength insufficient when learning Tai Chi. However, according to physiological principles, muscle contraction speed is directly proportional to the cube of energy consumption, so elderly or weak practitioners can reduce energy expenditure by using a higher stance and slowing down appropriately. The key issue here depends on the energy consumed by the large leg muscle groups. The combination of posture height and speed can greatly affect energy consumption, which can serve as a basis for selecting and examining exercise intensity.

However, is slower always better? The answer is no. The slowness of Tai Chi movement is relative to other martial arts. If the movement speed is too slow, it will inevitably cause breathing to become disconnected from the movements. The sayings "move energy as if drawing silk" and "step like a cat" simply emphasize that Tai Chi movements should be soft, continuous, sinking, and even, not that slower is always better. Moreover, slow movements can only avoid stiffness and rigidity when based on relaxation, tranquility, lightness, and softness. Otherwise, they may cause unnecessary tension in the nerves and muscles.

What is the appropriate slowness? It is when, in a calm and relaxed state of operation, one feels that the energy flows smoothly throughout the body, and the muscles and joints receive a gentle, beneficial functional stimulation. The appropriate speed must also vary according to one's physical condition and level of skill. For example, those with weaker constitutions who are just beginning to practice should use a higher stance, breathe naturally, and move more slowly, which helps with memorization and grasping key points, making it easier to use intention to guide movement. As skill deepens and physical condition improves, both fast and slow practice become possible. A set of simplified Tai Chi generally takes 4-7 minutes, which can be extended to 8-9 minutes for slow practice. The 88-form, Wu style, and Yang style Tai Chi are suitable at 10-25 minutes. Wu (Hao) style and Sun style Tai Chi are suitable at around 6-15 minutes. Chen style Tai Chi is suitable at around 5-8 minutes. However, it must be pointed out that speed differences can be quite significant based on personal preferences and practice requirements. For instance, some advocate that Wu or Yang style Tai Chi should take 50 minutes to complete a set, which cannot be considered incorrect.

Most Tai Chi styles advocate for uniform speed, with only Chen style Tai Chi incorporating elastic explosive force within the uniform speed. Tai Chi emphasizes slow and steady exercise of all body parts, which is a good method for elderly or weak individuals to develop or maintain physical strength evenly. However, practicing at a uniform speed also has its limitations: it cannot replace static exercises like standing post, nor does it include other dynamic exercises.

It must be noted that while Chen style Tai Chi includes moments of quick force generation, the uniform speed of other Tai Chi styles is relative to other forms of exercise and should not be seen as absolutely uniform. In practice, there is often a brief, almost imperceptible pause at the completion of each movement, marking the end of that movement, with intention and energy reaching to the fingertips, reinforcing stability, and providing a good start for the next movement. This creates a wave-like, alternating rhythm of tension and relaxation throughout the practice, reducing fatigue and maintaining a sense of mental clarity, enthusiasm, and reserve energy from beginning to end.

## 42. What is meant by "light, agile, sinking, and stable" and "hardness and softness complementing each other"?

Light means using intention, not force. Agile means circular and nimble movement. In the past, martial arts classics said: "Every movement of the whole body should be light and agile," but beginners should start with lightness first, without rushing to achieve agility. In other words, when starting to learn, focus on using as little force as possible under the guidance of intention, emphasizing lightness. After establishing a foundation in lightness, then work towards circular and nimble movements. Lightness is also the entry point for developing sensitive awareness.

Stability refers to practicing with a calm and composed spirit, and steady, grounded movements. Stability is achieved through mental calmness and full-body relaxation.

Tai Chi requires both lightness/agility and stability, so one must go through a period of practice to eliminate crude strength, moving from relaxation to softness.

What is softness? Softness means achieving controlled tension, maintaining appropriate tension while relaxing to the greatest extent possible. In other words, the muscle groups that should contract do so under the control of intention, while the antagonistic muscles relax in a timely manner, neither too late nor too early. Thus, hardness and softness are in some ways similar to emptiness and fullness. Softness is close to emptiness, hardness is close to fullness. After a period of practicing the transformation between emptiness and fullness in movements, the body can develop a state of "seeming relaxed but not relaxed," with "hardness and softness complementing each other," "combining lightness and stability, containing both hardness and softness." This results in firm, hard energy as well as elastic and resilient soft energy, extremely light and agile yet extremely stable, extremely soft yet extremely hard. However, at any given moment in a movement, hardness and softness are not equal. Looking at the overall practice, there is more time spent on softness than hardness. The process of each movement should be relaxed and gentle, only becoming hard at the moment of completion. But hardness and softness cannot be completely separated. The state of "seeming relaxed but not relaxed" is an internal energy that is neither soft nor hard, but can be either; "about to extend but not yet extended" is a state of potential energy, ready to be released. Chen style Tai Chi has visible external hard releases of energy (but still maintains elasticity and resilience); the 88-form, Yang, Sun, Wu (Hao), Wu, and Simplified Tai Chi styles only have an internal gathering of whole-body energy to a point at the moment of completion. Thus, some describe Tai Chi as "soft through the movement, hard at the point of completion," or "99% soft, 1% hard." Especially when practicing for health purposes, movements must emphasize relaxation and softness. In a state of mental calmness and concentration, using intention to guide movement, if one can relax the muscles and joints and move with light agility and stability, the qi and blood will flow smoothly, and long-term persistence will naturally benefit health. This prevents the development of stiff force in form practice or push hands, allowing for skillful changes and effective energy release in push hands.

How can one quickly master lightness, agility, stability, and the balance of hardness and softness?

1. First, practice with a relaxed mind and pay attention to relaxing the body.

2. Strictly follow the principle of "using intention, not force" in every movement. For visible hard releases of energy, don't use full force when practicing; start with 60-70% and gradually increase to 100%. If increasing force feels stiff and loses elasticity, without "circular liveliness," it indicates too much force is being used, and one should return to practicing with less force.

3. Coordinating movements with breathing helps develop lightness and agility during inhalation, and stability during exhalation.

4. When practicing forms, maintain "emptiness at the top of the head" (containing lightness and agility) and "relaxation or sinking qi to the lower abdomen" (containing stability). Raise the spirit as if floating on water, light above and sinking below, buoyant without sinking. "Clear spirit, sinking qi, naturally floating and bobbing in the waves, no matter how the wind and waves push, light above and sinking below, never toppling." This describes the state of being light above and sinking below during practice.

5. After mastering Tai Chi forms, practice two-person push hands to gradually experience the effects of lightness, agility, stability, and the balance of hardness and softness in movement.

## 43. What is the Significance of Circular and Spiral Movements in Tai Chi Chuan.

Tai Chi Chuan is characterized by its upper limb movements that often adopt circular, arc-shaped, or spiral forms (including small circles, large circles, ellipses, semicircles, and spatial curvilinear rotations). This approach is markedly different from the direct linear movements found in other martial arts. The complex and varied structure of Tai Chi Chuan, coupled with its graceful postures, is a result of generations of innovation and evolution.

Historically, the circular and arc-shaped movements in Tai Chi have been interpreted through metaphysical concepts such as the Taiji diagram, the Five Elements, the Bagua, and the principles of mutual generation and overcoming. Below, we explore these movements from physiological and push hands perspectives.

From a physiological standpoint, it is essential to understand that the body's joints (including the shoulders, elbows, wrists, hips, knees, and ankles) are spherical, resembling ball-and-socket joints, which ensure flexible movement. The body's movements are naturally diverse, with circular motions being the most natural due to the spherical structure of these joints. For instance, a movement originating from the shoulder joint, with the arm extended, naturally forms a circle. This is because such movements align with the joint's spherical anatomy. Beyond the major joints, the spine also comprises many smaller joints. The various circular, arc-shaped, and spiral movements of Tai Chi Chuan provide comprehensive exercise and balanced development for these numerous joints and engage multiple muscle groups. Movements like "Cloud Hands," "Repulse Monkey," and "Parting Wild Horse's Mane" involve almost every muscle in the body to different extents, facilitating the return flow of venous blood to the heart. Furthermore, the complex variations in circular movements effectively train the central nervous system, gradually enhancing its regulatory functions over all bodily organs.

In the context of push hands, circular or spiral movements are dynamically flexible and smooth, allowing for diverse changes that can neutralize and redirect an opponent's force in accordance with mechanical principles. The forces utilized in push hands encompass principles of levers, axles, force couples, resultant forces, centers of gravity, functions, and momentum, enabling a smaller force to overcome a larger one. Additionally, circular or spiral movements can adapt to any minor twist of the body, allowing for quick adjustments in technique (with minimal change in angle), which makes these movements effective both offensively and defensively. The ability to turn a disadvantageous position into a dominant one in push hands stems from the capability to utilize these circular movements across various joints. Thus, the distinctive circular and spiral movements in Tai Chi Chuan are not only a core aspect of its physical execution but also enhance its effectiveness and philosophical depth.

## 44. Why is Tai Chi Chuan Also Known as the Thirteen Postures?

According to traditional interpretations, the term "Thirteen Postures" in Tai Chi Chuan refers to the combination of the Five Elements and the Eight Trigrams. The Five Elements—metal, wood, water, fire, and earth—symbolize the five stepping methods in Tai Chi Chuan, while the Eight Trigrams—Qian (Heaven), Kun (Earth), Kan (Water), Li (Fire), Xun (Wind), Zhen (Thunder), Dui (Lake), and Gen (Mountain)—represent the eight hand techniques of the art.

In Tai Chi Chuan, the five steps consist of moving forward, backward, looking left, looking right (originally referring to eye movements but here interpreted as stepping actions), and centering oneself. The eight hand techniques are Ward Off (Peng), Roll Back (Lu), Press (Ji), Push (An), Pluck (Cai), Split (Lie), Elbow (Zhou), and Shoulder Strike (Kao), and they correspond to eight directions: east, west, south, north, northeast, northwest, southeast, and southwest. Together, these eight directions and five steps are collectively known as the Thirteen Postures, representing thirteen techniques rather than thirteen static poses.

Historically, the concepts of the "Five Elements" and "Eight Trigrams" carried with them a form of primitive materialist philosophy. However, given the limitations of historical conditions and the absence of modern scientific verification, these ideas were largely intuitive and speculative. While the five stepping methods and eight hand techniques in martial arts do exhibit dynamic interrelationships and contradictions, it must be acknowledged that applying the "Five Elements" and "Eight Trigrams" directly to Tai Chi Chuan today is not sufficiently scientific or comprehensive. For instance, the energetic pathways of techniques like Ward Off, Roll Back, Press, Push, Pluck, Split, Elbow, and Shoulder Strike cannot be fully depicted by a simple two-dimensional Bagua diagram; a three-dimensional coordinate system would be more scientifically appropriate. Additionally, it is not entirely accurate to rigidly assign the four primary techniques to the cardinal directions and the other four to the intercardinal directions, as, for example, the Shoulder Strike technique includes forward and backward applications, not just sideways. Therefore, it is essential to guide the practice of Tai Chi Chuan with a scientific dialectical materialist approach, employing modern scientific methods to study and organize the discipline effectively.

# Chapter Two

## Physiological Hygiene in Tai Chi Chuan Practice

### 1. What kind of environment is suitable for practicing Tai Chi Chuan?

The ideal setting for practicing Tai Chi Chuan is in an environment that offers abundant sunlight, fresh air, flat ground, and tranquility, whether outdoors or indoors. Practicing under sunlight has numerous benefits, including increased exposure to ultraviolet rays. Generally, it is preferable to practice when the sun is slanting rather than at its peak. During summer, those with weaker health should avoid practicing under direct sunlight and instead opt for shaded areas that still receive light.

The fresher the air, the better. Air pollution, which can include high levels of carbon dioxide, smoke, dust, and bacteria, is detrimental to health when inhaled into the lungs.

Beginners and those with weaker health or illnesses should practice on flat, spacious grounds to ensure stability. However, for those more adept, uneven ground can also be suitable as it benefits foot adaptability and enhances pushing hands techniques.

A quiet environment facilitates concentration and emotional calmness, which is especially important for beginners who are more easily distracted by external stimuli. If a quiet location is not available, one should aim to find tranquility amidst noise, a skill that can be developed over time.

Additionally, group practice can be synchronized with music, which helps maintain orderly movements and clear rhythm, benefiting beginners.

There is a notion that practicing Tai Chi Chuan in foggy weather is harmful to health, which requires specific analysis. Fog consists of water vapor that has condensed into tiny droplets near the ground. Practicing Tai Chi in areas where the air is fresh but foggy does not adversely affect health.

However, practicing in areas with heavy smoke and exhaust fumes is generally inadvisable. Fog in such polluted areas can worsen air quality by preventing the dispersion and dilution of pollutants, thus, it is essential to avoid practicing Tai Chi in polluted segments during foggy conditions.

## 2. When are the Optimal Times for Daily Tai Chi Practice?

Practicing Tai Chi Chuan is most beneficial at dawn or dusk. Morning practice capitalizes on the fresh air and tranquil environment, transitioning the body from a restful, inhibited state to an active state, energizing various organ functions and preparing the mind and body for the day's activities. In the evening, after a day's work, if one does not feel excessively fatigued, practicing Tai Chi can help alleviate physical and mental fatigue.

However, a disadvantage of practicing during these times is the lack of sunlight, which means missing out on the benefits of exercising in sunlight.

If practicing at these ideal times is not possible, one should tailor their exercise schedule to fit their personal circumstances. Practicing Tai Chi during work breaks can also be beneficial, especially for those engaged in mental labor, as it not only provides physical activity but also helps alleviate mental fatigue, which can be beneficial for productivity.

Similarly, physical laborers can benefit from moving during breaks to help eliminate fatigue and promote overall physical development.

Shift workers, including those on rotating shifts, can also achieve beneficial effects on their physical health by scheduling regular Tai Chi practice. For those starting early shifts, practicing in the early morning when possible allows for more vigorous activity; alternatively, practice can occur in the afternoon or evening, but not too late to avoid overstimulating the cerebral cortex and disrupting sleep.

For those on mid-day shifts, it is best to practice after 8:30 AM with a moderate level of activity.

For night shifts, practicing around 4:30 PM is advisable, with a lighter level of activity.

In summary, the timing of Tai Chi practice should be adapted to individual needs, times, and circumstances. If it is not possible to dedicate a continuous block of time, breaking the practice into several shorter sessions can also be effective.

## 3. How should one Gauge the Correct Exercise Intensity in Tai Chi Chuan Practice?

The appropriate exercise intensity in Tai Chi Chuan encompasses various factors including the duration of each session, the number of routines performed, the height of the stances, and the speed of execution. Exercise intensity should be tailored to the individual.

**How can one determine if the exercise intensity is appropriate?** A straightforward method is to perform a self-assessment of physical condition. Here are a couple of ways to conduct this assessment:

## Post-Practice Assessment:

If one notices improvement in conditions such as illness symptoms, mental state, appetite, and sleep quality after practicing Tai Chi, then the exercise intensity is likely appropriate. If body fatigue and soreness have largely subsided by the next morning, this also indicates a suitable exercise intensity. However, an absence of improvement or lingering soreness might suggest excessive practice.

Another morning check involves measuring your pulse upon waking and comparing it with the previous day. If there is no significant change, or if the pulse has slowed down gradually, the exercise intensity might be insufficient and could be moderately increased or maintained.

## Fatigue Monitoring:

A simple way to manage exercise intensity is to adhere to the traditional principle often summarized by laborers: "Do not exhaust yourself with practice." Fatigue is an important signal indicating that both the brain and heart require rest. Therefore, as a means of therapy, it is advisable to stop practicing when slightly fatigued to prevent overexertion.

If one is highly engaged and interested in practicing, fatigue may be delayed, and it is advisable to perform the aforementioned checks during such times. Ending practice while still feeling enthusiastic can be very effective. If one feels energetic and refreshed after finishing the session, it generally indicates an appropriate exercise intensity that has optimally benefited physical fitness.

Healthy individuals without illnesses can practice for about an hour each day. Beginners and those with weaker constitutions should adjust the exercise intensity based on their physical condition. They may perform a single routine or several, focus on individual sections or specific movements such as "Grasping the Sparrow's Tail" or "Cloud Hands." An effective way to increase the exercise intensity is to lower the stance height. Those with weaker health should start with higher stances and, as they gain proficiency and strength, gradually transition to medium or low stances. Different injuries or illnesses require adjustments in the exercise intensity and method of practice.

## 4. What should be the Guidelines for Practicing Tai Chi Chuan for Individuals with Weakness or Chronic Illness?

Individuals with weakness or chronic illness should tailor their Tai Chi Chuan practice to their physical condition and health status, considering the appropriate timing, frequency, and intensity of exercise. Here, some general principles are offered for reference, with specific conditions requiring consultation of specialized topics.

### Medical Supervision:

Patients in hospitals or sanatoriums should practice under the guidance of a physician.

### Consistency and Persistence:

Practicing Tai Chi Chuan must be done consistently and for the long term. Many patients, eager for a quick cure, hope to recover within a few days. Others lack determination and confidence, practicing only sporadically when they have free time or feel inclined. Such an inconsistent approach yields poor results. The benefits of Tai Chi Chuan on the body develop gradually, often taking two to three months before noticeable improvement or recovery is seen. Experience has shown that individuals without illnesses who persistently practice can enhance their physical health, increase vitality, and experience fewer illnesses.

## Gradual Progression:

The timing of practice, the intensity of exercise, and the difficulty of movements should be gradually increased, tailored to individual capabilities. Excessive exercise can lead to overtiredness. If proficiency has been achieved, symptoms have lessened, and physical strength has improved, then it is appropriate to gradually increase the exercise intensity and complexity to continuously improve health levels.

## Alternating Exercise and Rest:

Exercise and rest should alternate. During each exercise session, take short breaks based on personal stamina.

## Monitoring Post-Exercise Responses:

Pay close attention to how the body reacts after exercising to gauge if the exercise intensity is appropriate. Generally, it is normal for the pulse to increase by 20-40 beats per minute during exercise, accompanied by mild fatigue, which should dissipate a few minutes after resting.

After exercising, one should feel comfortable and refreshed. If the pulse increases significantly during exercise, leading to extreme fatigue, or if physical strength does not recover even after a long rest, and symptoms like palpitations, shortness of breath, loss of appetite, or poor sleep occur, these indicate that the exercise intensity is too high. In such cases, it is advisable to reduce the exercise intensity or take appropriate rest. If there are no adverse reactions and health continues to improve, then gradually increasing the exercise intensity and difficulty can be beneficial.

## 5. What preparations should be made before practicing Tai Chi?

Before practicing Tai Chi Chuan, it is essential to prepare the body to relax the muscles and tendons, loosen the joints, expand the lungs, and ensure blood circulation. Begin with a light walk, followed by movements that involve the limbs and torso, such as bending over to stretch the legs, performing standing postures, and doing several deep breaths. Also, practice some key Tai Chi movements like "Cloud Hands," "Part Wild Horse's Mane," and "Grasping the Sparrow's Tail" individually. Since Tai Chi Chuan is a gentle form of exercise, the physical warm-up does not need to be intense—three to five minutes is generally sufficient.

Mental preparation is also crucial for practicing Tai Chi Chuan. The art requires a calm mind and focused spirit. To achieve this, you can slightly open your eyes or gaze into the distance before beginning, focus on calming the mind, and relax each joint sequentially from head to toe until the entire body feels relaxed and the spirit is serene, fostering a peaceful and harmonious state.

## 6. What should one Do After Completing a Tai Chi Chuan Session?

After finishing a Tai Chi Chuan session, it is important to maintain the same mental focus as during practice. Slowly walk around for three to five minutes before resuming normal activities. This approach has two main benefits:

### Physiological Transition:

During Tai Chi practice, breathing deepens and blood circulation accelerates, with all physiological functions in a heightened state of activity. Slow walking after finishing helps these physiological activities gradually ease back to their normal pace, facilitating a smooth transition back to resting conditions.

### Mental and Neurological Benefits:

While practicing Tai Chi, the mind is focused and the cerebral cortex undergoes a series of functional adjustments, inducing numerous beneficial physiological responses and conditioned reflexes. These responses and connections continue even after the session ends. Allowing them to taper off slowly helps to solidify and enhance the positive effects of these responses.

## 7. What to do if your legs feel sore when learning Tai Chi Chuan?

Leg soreness is common for beginners in Tai Chi Chuan, largely due to the need for the legs to alternately bear the body's weight either partially or fully, and the requirement to bend the legs while transitioning slowly between positions. This significantly increases the load on the lower limb muscles, leading to soreness.

Consistent and prolonged practice can strengthen the heart, improve blood circulation, increase lung capacity, and consequently reduce muscle soreness. Even when the exercise intensity is high, the soreness will be mild and recovery will be quicker.

To minimize soreness, consider the following tips:

### Adequate Warm-up:

Perform proper warm-up exercises before starting your Tai Chi routine.

### Gradual Increase in Exercise Intensity:

Adjust the exercise intensity based on personal physical condition and gradually increase it.

### Cool-down Activities:

Engage in cool-down activities, such as slow walking, after practicing Tai Chi.

### Relief Measures:

If experiencing intense soreness, consider applying heat locally with a towel, soaking the feet in warm water, taking a warm bath, massaging the sore areas with your hands, or using topical applications like camphor spirit or pine oil.

Muscle soreness is not a pathological condition but a normal physiological response. With continued practice, this phenomenon will naturally diminish.

## 8. Can one Practice Tai Chi Chuan During Menstruation, Pregnancy, and Lactation?

### Menstruation:

Generally, healthy women can continue practicing Tai Chi Chuan during their menstrual period. Proper activity not only does not interfere with the normal menstrual cycle but can also improve pelvic blood circulation, reduce pelvic congestion, shorten the duration of the period, and help regulate brain functions related to excitement and inhibition. Consequently, it can alleviate symptoms like lower back pain, bloating, a sensation of heaviness in the lower abdomen, or mood disturbances. The intensity of exercise should be adjusted based on personal comfort, either reduced slightly or maintained as usual.

## Pregnancy:

Engaging in gentle Tai Chi Chuan exercises during pregnancy is beneficial. However, certain poses (such as deep squats, Golden Rooster Stands on One Leg, Needle at Sea Bottom, and separate leg stances) should be avoided in the later stages of pregnancy. Practicing simpler movements like "Cloud Hands" or "Parting Wild Horse's Mane" can be advantageous. Sun exposure during exercise can help convert dehydrocholesterol in the skin into vitamin D, which aids in the absorption and utilization of calcium and phosphorus—minerals that are crucial during pregnancy. Outdoor practice can be beneficial for both maternal and fetal health by supplementing calcium and phosphorus, reducing pre-delivery symptoms like edema and constipation, and facilitating smoother childbirth. Exercise during pregnancy should be cautious, especially close to delivery, and conducted under medical supervision.

## Lactation:

During lactation, appropriate Tai Chi Chuan practice in sunlight can aid postnatal physical recovery and increase the calcium and phosphorus content in breast milk. It is advisable to pause Tai Chi practice during the immediate postpartum period and engage in postnatal therapeutic exercises under medical guidance.

# 9. How Should One Manage Their Diet When Practicing Tai Chi Chuan?

Tai Chi Chuan movements are generally gentle, and it's common to practice on an empty stomach early in the morning without eating beforehand. However, practicing on an empty stomach can cause some individuals to feel hungry, and with a significant amount of exercise, it may lead to symptoms such as dizziness, palpitations, and weakness. These symptoms are typically due to low blood sugar levels. If these symptoms occur, it is advisable to stop practicing immediately and drink a sugary beverage. Therefore, for those who are frail, it is best not to practice too long before breakfast, ideally keeping to about 30 minutes to an hour.

After practicing Tai Chi Chuan, especially an intense session like those of Chen style, the body remains in an excited state. Some people may find their appetite is poor right after exercise; it is optimal to wait about 10 to 20 minutes before eating.

Practicing Tai Chi soon after eating can be uncomfortable as the gastrointestinal tract is full, causing discomfort from the food moving back and forth during the exercise. The human body has about 2-3 liters of circulating blood, which is not evenly distributed but directed where it is most needed. After eating, blood vessels in the digestive organs such as the stomach, intestines, and pancreas dilate significantly for digestion, increasing blood flow, enhancing function, and boosting secretion levels. The pancreas secretes insulin and pancreatic juice, aiding in the digestion of carbohydrates, fats, and proteins. During physical activity, the blood vessels in the limbs dilate extensively to support active muscles, ligaments, and joints, which increases blood flow to these areas. Conversely, the blood supply to the digestive organs decreases, reducing digestive capacity. Therefore, it is not advisable to practice Tai Chi immediately after eating. It is best to wait at least half an hour before beginning to practice.

## 10. Is It Correct to Avoid Urination or Defecation Before Morning Tai Chi Practice?

There is an old belief that one should not urinate or defecate before morning exercise, as it supposedly "drains energy" and prevents the attainment of "true skill." This notion has no scientific basis.

From a physiological perspective, nutrients from food provide energy for various bodily functions. After digestion in the gastrointestinal tract, the absorbed nutrients leave behind residues that form feces. Excess water in the body, along with waste products from the metabolism of muscles, tissues, and blood, are excreted by the kidneys as urine. Before elimination, urine and feces are stored in the bladder and rectum, respectively, and no longer participate in physiological activities but are merely waste waiting to be expelled. Therefore, retaining them does not benefit physical performance. On the contrary, it is advisable to empty the bladder and bowels before exercising (deliberately holding in the need to urinate or defecate at any time is harmful). This not only reduces the physical burden and relieves unnecessary tension during Tai Chi practice but also prevents potential injuries, such as a bladder rupture during push hands, and avoids constipation.

Ignoring the urge to defecate can lead to chronic constipation. Over time, the rectum may stop responding to the need to evacuate, contributing to constipation, which can cause pelvic organ venous congestion and provoke conditions like hemorrhoids. This is particularly impactful for women, potentially affecting menstrual functions (irregular menstruation, painful periods) and causing uterine misalignment. If the rectum is overly distended, it can push the cervix forward, causing the uterus to tilt backward due to the lever principle. An over-distended or infrequently emptied bladder can also cause a backward tilt of the uterus. If this condition recurs over a long period, the veins in the broad ligaments may become compressed and obstructed, leading to congestion in the uterine wall, loss of elasticity, and chronic pain in the sacral region, lower back pain, and menstrual disorders.

## 11. Why Do Some People's Hands Get Cold After Practicing Tai Chi in Winter?"

The human body's organs and tissues differ in their heat production, blood supply, and the rate at which they release heat, resulting in varying temperatures. For example, the liver, due to its robust metabolism, generates a lot of heat, often reaching temperatures of about 38°C or higher. Similarly, the temperature across different parts of the body surface varies; generally, the head and face have higher temperatures, followed by the chest and abdomen, with the extremities being the coldest. The limbs, having a large surface area, dissipate heat quickly, and during Tai Chi practice, the hands are exposed and lose heat the fastest. Thus, it's normal for some people to have warm hands before practicing Tai Chi in winter, but find them cold afterward. If only one hand becomes cold, this could be due to individual differences such as uneven sweating, different body temperatures on each side, or more relaxed movement in one hand (often the right). If there are no other symptoms of discomfort, it is generally not a concern. For instance, there was a person who practiced Tai Chi for many decades and always had one hand warmer than the other after practice, yet he lived healthily into his nineties.

Moreover, it's important to note that individuals who undergo cold-weather training tend to have higher skin temperatures in their limbs compared to those who do not train, with no significant difference in trunk temperature. Practicing Tai Chi outdoors in winter effectively enhances the body's adaptability to natural environments and increases cold resistance, serving as a preventative measure against frostbite in the limbs. Relaxing the body during practice, focusing energy at the fingertips in the final stance (ensuring energy reaches the extremities), and properly executing techniques like sinking the shoulders and dropping the elbows, as well as settling the wrists, can improve blood circulation in the extremities. This often helps overcome the issue of cold hands, and some practitioners even experience a warm and comfortable feeling after practice.

## 12. What Causes Shaking During Tai Chi Practice and How to Prevent It?

Shaking during Tai Chi practice, especially during certain twisting movements (like Cloud Hands and High Pat on Horse) or strenuous activities (such as Golden Rooster Stands on One Leg and separate leg stances), is a common issue that can vary in intensity and may seem uncontrollable. This shaking usually occurs because many people are not accustomed to the light and agile movements characteristic of Tai Chi. Tension and failure to relax the muscles, particularly during rotational movements, are frequent contributors to this problem. Beginners are especially prone to this issue. Some practitioners may not experience shaking during regular practice but find themselves trembling during competitions or performances due to increased tension. Others might mistakenly believe that shaking is a positive sign, indicating that "energy is being stimulated" and that their skills have reached a certain level, thus they might even intentionally cultivate this shaking.

It's important to clarify that shaking is not a normal phenomenon nor an indication of skill development in Tai Chi; rather, it is a flaw and deviation.

To prevent this issue, practitioners should aim to keep their mind calm and their muscles relaxed, without any tension during practice. Movements should be natural and spontaneous, with hand extensions and changes in posture occurring effortlessly. The learning process should be gradual and not rushed. Adhering to these principles can help correct the occurrence of unintentional shaking. If the habit of shaking has already developed, it is crucial to make a concerted effort to correct it. Like a beginner, one should focus on rectifying this flaw in every movement, which can eventually lead to improvement.

## 13. Is it good to make sounds while practicing Tai chi Chuan? What is the impact of talking while practicing?

Making occasional natural sounds during Tai Chi practice, especially during push hands or when exerting force, can enhance the overall power of the movements. This is because vocalizing tends to tense the abdominal muscles, which coordinates with the tension in the back muscles and the natural contraction of the rib cage (chest ribs moving forward and down), strengthening the solid effect of the exhalation during the exertion. Historically, martial artists have cataloged various sounds such as eight sounds (Peng, Ye, Xi, Ke, Hu, Hang, He, Ha), six sounds (Zhao, He, Hu, Xu, Chui, Xi), five sounds (Xu, He, Shen, Chui, Hu), four sounds (Ha, Ke, Yi, Wei), three sounds (Heng, Ha, Ke), and two sounds (Heng, Ha). These are the experiences of past practitioners, warranting further exploration.

Based on the compiler's experience, the sound "Hei" is particularly useful for deepening the stance, increasing the elasticity and explosive force of the arm movements. The "Hei" sound can be made loudly or softly. For therapeutic purposes, the sound "He" is more effective, aiding in the downward movement of Qi and blood. However, the "He" sound should be as long as the exhalation, and the vocalization should not be loud, just perceivable to the practitioner.

Whether using "Hei" or "He," these sounds are made occasionally during exhalation. The "He" sound can be continuously integrated six or seven times.

Talking while practicing Tai Chi disrupts the natural depth and rhythm of breathing and breaks the concentration necessary for effective practice, thereby diminishing the benefits of the exercise. Therefore, it is best to avoid talking while practicing.

## 14. How Should We View the Concept of "Promoting Longevity and Eternal Youth" in Tai Chi Chuan?

The old saying in martial arts discourse, "What ultimately is the purpose of pushing hands? To promote longevity and eternal youth," was once considered an unattainable ideal in old societies. In those times, the working people, exploited by the ruling classes, struggled with basic necessities like sufficient food and warm clothing, let alone aspiring for "longevity and eternal youth." Today, under a socialist society, this phrase should be analyzed from a proletarian perspective. Nowadays, our ethos is "not to fear hardship nor death," aiming to contribute bravely to the socialist and communist revolution.

The desires for extended life and "philosophy of survival" represent the ideologies of the exploiting classes and should be eradicated from the Tai Chi Chuan community. Our purpose in practicing Tai Chi is to extend our productive years for the socialist revolution and construction, and to enhance work efficiency. When the revolution calls for sacrifices, we should be prepared to give our all courageously. However, we should minimize unnecessary sacrifices. The body is a resource for the revolution, and it is incorrect not to actively train and protect it. Nevertheless, physical training is not for survival but for the revolution.

If our elderly can extend their working years and maintain their revolutionary vigor and skills, imagine the immense contributions they could make to our socialist revolution and construction! However, it is crucial to note that just like attaining a healthy body, "promoting longevity and eternal youth" is not something predestined or bestowed; it must be fought for and earned through persistent and serious training. Practice has shown that consistent Tai Chi practice can indeed play a role in preventing premature aging. Under the wise leadership of Chairman Mao and the Party Central Committee, and within our superior socialist system, the aspiration of "promoting longevity and eternal youth" is achievable in our country.

## 15. Is it possible to practice other physical activities while learning Tai Chi Chuan?

This query has historically sparked considerable debate, leading to two conflicting viewpoints.

One perspective holds that practicing Tai Chi Chuan precludes the simultaneous practice of Long Fist, free sparring, and exercises like parallel bars, citing the unique nature of energy and force utilized in Tai Chi compared to other sports. Tai Chi advocates for the principle of using 'intention' rather than brute strength, contrasting sharply with the force-driven techniques of Long Fist and free sparring. Proponents of this view argue that practicing both concurrently can lead to a compromise in mastering either, especially for beginners. Struggling to switch between the subtle use of 'intention' in Tai Chi and the overt use of force in other disciplines can lead to inefficacy at best, and internal injuries at worst. This assertion, however, lacks scientific substantiation and often stems from historical socio-cultural dynamics where martial arts were monopolized by ruling classes to preserve their status, leading to the propagation of exclusivity and mystification.

Conversely, the second viewpoint supports the concurrent practice of different martial arts or physical disciplines. Advocates believe that with proper training and appropriate scheduling, a practitioner can reap the benefits of both rigid and flexible forms. For example, practicing Long Fist could enhance one's firmness and strength, while Tai Chi could cultivate suppleness and fluidity. A practitioner skilled in both could achieve a balance, embodying the best of both worlds, thereby facilitating easier victories in combat through a deeper understanding of both hard and soft techniques.

I align with this latter viewpoint, provided several considerations are observed:

## For beginners:

It is advisable not to engage in different styles of physical activities simultaneously within the same period. Structuring one's training schedule—perhaps practicing one discipline in the morning and another in the afternoon or on alternate days—can be more beneficial. Once a solid foundation in each practice is established, simultaneous training becomes more feasible.

## Moderation is key:

Regardless of the number of disciplines practiced, overtraining must be avoided to prevent excessive physical fatigue and consequent health detriment. Each activity should be pursued within one's physical limits to maintain overall health and well-being.

## 16. Why do people with neurasthenia benefit significantly from practicing Tai Chi Chuan, and what should they be mindful of?

Neurasthenia is characterized by a cluster of symptoms primarily indicating an imbalance between the excitatory and inhibitory processes of the cerebral cortex, without any organic changes to the body. This condition, rooted in excessive worry, prolonged negative psychological factors, overly tense emotions, and an imbalance between work and life that excludes appropriate physical or manual activity, leads to a disruption in the basic functions of cerebral excitation and inhibition. This imbalance reduces the brain's regulatory and directive functions on the body, manifesting as insomnia, dizziness, and weakened memory.

Practicing Tai Chi Chuan can play a positive role in the prevention and treatment of neurasthenia and other conditions caused by dysfunction of the nervous system. Tai Chi requires a dynamic balance between activity and stillness, demanding intense concentration and mental focus during practice. This focus induces a regular pattern of excitation in the parts of the cerebral cortex involved in movement, while allowing other areas to enter a state of inhibition and rest. This process is what we refer to as an "active rest" beneficial for the brain. Just as daily concentrated work excites specific brain cells related to that activity, practicing Tai Chi allows these overstimulated cells to rest and recuperate, often leaving practitioners feeling mentally refreshed and clear, as if their minds were cleansed with water.

Additionally, Tai Chi provides rigorous training and adjustment for brain function. The complex, engaging, and enjoyable movements of Tai Chi integrate mental, emotional, sensory, and physical aspects, creating a harmonious exercise experience. This not only trains the entire nervous system but continuously tunes and exercises the brain functions throughout the practice. Long-term adherence can significantly restore and enhance brain functions, as evidenced by numerous cases, including a senior comrade who overcame severe neurasthenia after practicing Tai Chi for a month following twenty years of ineffective treatments.

Key considerations for practitioners with neurasthenia:

### Exercise Moderation:

Start with lighter exercise volumes and gradually increase. If the exercise volume is appropriate, symptoms should diminish and recovery ensue.

### Manage Expectations:

Patients should avoid impatience and maintain faith in gradual improvement, rather than expecting instant recovery.

### Tailored Exercise Time:

Evening practice may aid sleep for some but hinder it for others. It's crucial to find a personal schedule that suits one's condition and does not disrupt sleep—perhaps exercising 2-4 hours before bedtime can improve sleep.

### Lifestyle Regularity:

A structured yet relaxed lifestyle is crucial. An unregulated life, even with full rest, can worsen the condition. Too much idle time can depress mental activity and mood, which can negatively impact disease treatment.

## 17. What should patients with pulmonary tuberculosis be aware of when practicing Tai Chi Chuan?

Tai Chi Chuan has been recognized for its significant therapeutic benefits in the treatment and consolidation of pulmonary tuberculosis. Post-liberation, many hospitals and sanatoriums across the country have affirmed that appropriately practiced Tai Chi Chuan can greatly assist in the comprehensive treatment of this disease. Tai Chi enhances the central nervous system's regulation of bodily functions, improves respiratory function, increases oxygen exchange, strengthens hematopoietic and mineral metabolism, positively impacts the autonomic nervous system, and boosts physiological immunity. This helps patients recover more quickly, prevents deterioration of the condition, or recurrence of the disease.

Previously, the treatment for pulmonary tuberculosis often involved bed rest, which inevitably hindered metabolic functions and weakened vitality. Therefore, except during periods of exacerbation where bed rest and other therapies are necessary, patients should engage in appropriate physical activities daily.

Ideal candidates for Tai Chi practice include:

1. Patients in the absorption or calcification phase of primary pulmonary tuberculosis or hilar lymph node tuberculosis.

2. Patients with recurrent chronic pulmonary tuberculosis entering the absorption or consolidation phase, where clinical symptoms have subsided, no fever is present, sedimentation rate is normal or slightly elevated (not exceeding 30 mm in the first hour), no hemoptysis, and no adverse reactions after activities.

3. Patients with chronic fibrocavernous pulmonary tuberculosis in a stable condition, even if cavities are present in the lungs.

During the initial stages of practicing Tai Chi, patients may experience increased sputum and pulse rate, which typically decrease and disappear shortly thereafter. Some debilitated patients might find the initial practice intolerable, but if lab tests, X-rays, and scans show no changes in the lesions and no adverse bodily reactions, the practice should not be discontinued out of fear; rather, the exercise volume should be reduced.

Positive indications to continue practicing include:

1. A pulse increase that diminishes as practice progresses.

2. Gradual reduction in pulmonary inflammation.

3. Reduction or disappearance of cough.

4. Alleviation or disappearance of asthma.

5. Weight stabilization or increase.

6. A decrease in neutrophil band forms and an increase in lymphocytes.

7. Absorption of new infiltrative lesions.

Practice should be discontinued if any of the following adverse conditions occur:

1. Increase in body temperature.

2. Increase in sedimentation rate.

3. Significant increase in cough and expectoration, accompanied by respiratory distress.

4. Substantial hemoptysis.

5. X-ray evidence of worsening condition.

6. Significant acceleration of pulse.

7. Weight loss.

8. Increase in neutrophil band forms and decrease in lymphocytes.

Patients should not practice Tai Chi if there is X-ray evidence of progressing lung changes, increased infiltration, or cavity formation, even if clinical symptoms appear normal and there are no adverse reactions after activities. Also, those with highly increased sedimentation rates, persistent fever, or frequent recent hemoptysis should refrain from practicing.

Patients with the following conditions should not practice Tai Chi:

1. Active hilar lymph node tuberculosis.

2. Exacerbation phase of exudative pleurisy.

3. Tuberculous peritonitis.

4. Active mesenteric lymph node tuberculosis.

5. Ulcerative bronchial tuberculosis.

6. Bone tuberculosis.

7. Active genitourinary tuberculosis.

### Practice recommendations:

Movements should be gentle and slow, without rigid force. Natural breathing techniques should be adopted, and exercise volume should gradually increase. Practice duration should be about 15-30 minutes per session, once or twice a day, tailored to the patient's condition. In sanatoriums, group practices can be organized into light, medium, and heavy activity groups based on patient condition.

Furthermore, practicing in a pine or cypress forest, if feasible, can be particularly beneficial as these trees emit phytoncides that have an inhibitory effect on tuberculosis bacteria.

## 18. Can people with bronchitis practice Tai Chi Chuan, and what should they be mindful of?

Bronchitis can generally be classified as acute or chronic. Acute bronchitis often presents symptoms such as fever, coughing, sticky phlegm, sore throat, and chest pain, and exercise should be avoided during onset. Chronic bronchitis often develops following acute bronchitis, and can also be caused by frequent colds, exposure to cold, excessive smoking, or poor working conditions. Regularly practicing Tai Chi is very beneficial for people with chronic bronchitis. Practicing Tai Chi can naturally deepen and lengthen breathing, directly exercising the respiratory organs, allowing the blood to combine with more oxygen in the lungs, and then transport it to tissue cells, ensuring better life activities of tissue cells. Combining medication and other treatments with persistent practice can improve blood and lymph circulation in the chest cavity, promote absorption of exudates in inflamed areas, and accelerate the improvement of bronchitis, but the following points should be noted during exercise.

Exercise and drug treatment should be coordinated. When the condition is stable, in addition to drug treatment, Tai Chi or medical gymnastics can be practiced to enhance the body's resistance and improve the efficacy of medication. If there is an acute exacerbation, appropriate rest and timely treatment are necessary.

When practicing Tai Chi, it is best to adopt natural deep breathing, but attention should be paid to prolonging the exhalation time, and nasal inhalation and exhalation should be used as much as possible. The amount of activity should not be too large.

In winter, the climate is cold and dry, and people with bronchitis have weak resistance of the respiratory mucosa and poor adaptation to cold. Once they catch a cold, it is easy to cause a recurrence of the old illness and aggravate symptoms. Those who are new to practicing should preferably start before the cold weather sets in.

Do not remove clothing too early before the body has warmed up during exercise, quickly put on outer clothing during exercise intervals and after exercise, and wipe off sweat. It is best to change out of wet clothes to avoid catching a cold.

## 19. How can one prevent catching a cold while practicing Tai Chi Chuan?

The common cold is an acute respiratory infectious disease caused by a filterable virus. Cold stimulation of the human body reduces the body's resistance, at which time the cold viruses hiding in the nasal cavity and throat become active, invade the trachea, causing inflammation of the mucous membranes of the nasal cavity, throat, and trachea, and even affecting the tonsils to become inflamed and swollen, thus producing a series of symptoms such as clear nasal discharge, sneezing, coughing, and sore throat. If it affects the vocal cords, it may also cause hoarseness. This is the common cold, also known as upper respiratory tract infection. Long-term persistence in outdoor Tai Chi practice or other exercises not only will not cause colds, but is actually an effective means of preventing colds. Some people occasionally catch colds during Tai Chi practice or other exercises, mainly due to lack of attention to hygiene during exercise. As long as you pay attention to the following points, Tai Chi practice or other exercises will not cause colds.

In winter, do not wear too little clothing when just going from indoors to outdoors, as the temperature difference between indoors and outdoors is large in winter. As you practice, the body gradually warms up, then remove thick clothing; by this time the body has already warmed up, making it less likely to catch a cold.

Furthermore, after sweating, dry your body in a windless indoor area, change out of wet clothes, and put on dry clothes; do not seek coolness by wearing sweat-soaked clothes in the wind, as this easily leads to catching a cold. Even if the underwear is not wet, you should promptly put on warm clothes after practicing to avoid catching a cold.

In addition, breathing should be correct during practice. Generally, nasal breathing should be used; if nasal inhalation is insufficient, you can slightly open your mouth, letting cold air enter through the gaps between teeth, breathing through both mouth and nose, avoiding direct stimulation of the throat by cold air which can cause a cold.

The amount of exercise should be appropriate, not too much. If the amount of exercise is too large, the body becomes overly fatigued, which can also lower resistance and lead to colds.

The main reason for catching a cold in summer is that the external temperature is high, and for better heat dissipation, the capillaries on the body surface are in a dilated state, with sweat pores all open. At this time, if one is not careful, such as seeking momentary coolness by taking a cold shower immediately after practice, or if a sudden cold wind or light rain comes after exercise, causing the body to suddenly cool down, it is easy to catch a cold. Therefore, after practicing in summer, you should also add or remove clothing in a timely manner according to weather changes, not take a cold shower immediately after exercise, wait until sweating has stopped before bathing, and put on clothes immediately after bathing. Especially when sweat has not dried and one seeks coolness in a drafty place, it often leads to colds or other illnesses.

In short, whether in winter, summer, spring, or autumn, paying attention to hygiene during practice will not cause colds.

Moreover, as long as one persists in practicing martial arts or other exercises, with the strengthening of physical fitness and the improvement of adaptability to the environment and resistance to pathogens, one can more effectively prevent colds.

## 20. Why is Tai Chi Chuan effective in preventing and treating heart disease, and what should heart patients be mindful of when practicing?

Heart disease patients, due to their low cardiac reserve, often experience palpitations and shortness of breath after activity, and may even develop heart failure. This often causes patients to rest. However, the longer one rests, the lower the overall body function becomes, especially cardiac reserve function. Once beyond this resting adaptation range, such as with slightly increased activity, infection or emotional excitement, heart failure can easily occur. Not to mention patients, even healthy people will gradually reduce heart function with prolonged bed rest. A heart research institute once conducted the following experiment. Several men aged 20-30 who were determined to be completely healthy by a special committee were required to lie down continuously for 20 days and nights according to the experiment's regulations, not allowed to sit up, stand or exercise. Another group for verification also followed these regulations, with the only difference being they could exercise four times a day on special equipment while maintaining a lying position. By 3-5 days into the experiment, all participants experienced muscle soreness, loss of appetite, and constipation. After 20 days and nights, when the participants stood up from bed, they felt dizzy, extremely weak muscles, and abnormally rapid pulse; many people's pulse became extremely weak rather than rapid after standing up, arterial pressure dropped to dangerous levels and they were in a fainting state; cardiac function decreased by 70%, tissues lacked oxygen; any activity (such as walking indoors) caused muscle pain, lasting until 2-4 days after the experiment ended. However, the verification group that exercised during the trial period maintained their working ability. This shows that insufficient activity can cause changes in the central nervous system and endocrine system, which in turn leads to emotional instability, metabolic disorders, muscle mass reduction, changes in bone tissue mineral saturation, drastic changes in the cardiovascular system, and gastrointestinal dysfunction.

From this, it can be seen that regular exercise and physical labor are important and effective means of strengthening the heart. The Sports Medicine Research Institute of Beijing Medical College found that regular Tai Chi practice also has beneficial effects on the cardiovascular system. Comparing elderly people who regularly practice Tai Chi with normal elderly people, both groups underwent a functional test (stepping up and down a 40 cm high bench 15 times in one minute). The results showed that the Tai Chi group had better cardiovascular function. Of the 32 elderly people, except for one who could not complete the specified load, the rest could all complete it, and their blood pressure and pulse response types were normal. In contrast, in the control group, the older the age, the fewer people could complete the specified load, and more people showed poor functional test response types (such as ladder-like ascending type and powerless type responses). Electrocardiogram examinations also proved this point. Abnormal ECG responses (such as prolonged P-R, QRS and QT intervals, decreased Rv5 wave amplitude, ST segment depression, T wave inversion, etc. after exercise) were only 28.2% in the Tai Chi group, while 41.3% in the control group of ordinary elderly people. From these observations, it is not difficult to see that regular Tai Chi practice can make coronary artery blood supply to the heart adequate, heart contraction strong, and blood dynamics good. In Tai Chi exercise, not only is there muscle tension and relaxation, but also spiral-shaped advancing, retreating and twisting, which promotes venous blood return more than general exercise; coupled with Tai Chi's ability to improve respiratory system function and increase chest and abdominal pressure changes, this also helps venous blood return to the heart, thus increasing the stroke volume of each heart contraction, which is beneficial for heart function.

The occurrence of heart disease requires certain conditions. For example, the occurrence of the most common coronary heart disease is generally a relatively slow process. Taking appropriate measures can prevent its occurrence or control its condition, maintain a certain working ability, and even be unaffected. The main reason for coronary artery hardening is the deposition of lipids in the arterial intima. The main component of lipids is cholesterol. Many people who regularly practice Tai Chi and participate in various physical exercises have significantly lower blood cholesterol levels than those who do not participate in activities, which directly reduces the pathogenic factors of atherosclerosis, playing a role of "removing the firewood from under the cauldron" in the pathogenesis. More importantly, long-term persistence in exercise increases the number of capillaries in the myocardium, causing small blood vessel branches on both sides of narrowed and obstructed coronary artery segments to dilate, interconnect, and establish collateral circulation. When collateral circulation is established, the blood supply to the heart improves, improving or eliminating symptoms.

In addition, practical evidence shows that most coronary heart disease patients can enjoy a full lifespan like normal people, with only a very small number eventually developing myocardial infarction. Even those who have had a myocardial infarction can regain partial work and life abilities with timely and appropriate treatment. Therefore, after getting coronary heart disease or other heart diseases, there is no need to be pessimistic, afraid to move all day, even bedridden all day, or blindly believe in medication. Of course, medication is one aspect of treatment, but "external causes are the conditions of change, internal causes are the basis of change, external causes work through internal causes." To make medication work well, one must mobilize the body's internal factors and enhance resistance. Appropriate participation in physical exercise is a powerful means of mobilizing internal factors.

Heart disease patients should pay attention to the following points when engaging in physical exercise:

1. Acute myocarditis, myocardial infarction or other heart diseases causing heart failure or acute angina attacks are not suitable for practicing Tai Chi.

2. The amount of exercise should be moderate, with slight fatigue. If there is slight palpitation or shortness of breath, this exercise session must be stopped. Because each patient's condition is different, it is necessary to grasp the right measure and overcome tendencies of fear of movement or blind movement. Some people, having tasted the sweetness of exercise, suddenly increase their activity level, causing unfavorable situations, which should be avoided. Appropriate rest is still necessary for patients with more severe heart disease. For heart disease patients who experience sudden circulatory failure, special care should be taken in handling, as even slight exertion can quickly cause breathlessness, palpitations, and congestion in various parts of the body. Such

patients should initially perform lying or sitting medical exercises, and after improvement, gradually engage in Tai Chi exercise, starting with practicing a few single movements and gradually increasing the amount of exercise as the condition improves.

3. Try to maintain regular daily life, avoid emotional fluctuations such as anger and sorrow, arrange work reasonably, have sufficient sleep time (but not too much), and have appropriate compensatory rest after intense,□□□ work.

4. The total calorie intake in the diet should not be too high, aiming to maintain body weight at the level of [height (cm) - 100 = weight (kg)] or thereabouts. Some people pay attention to not eating animal fats and high-cholesterol foods, but have excessive sugar and total calorie intake, which can lead to high blood neutral fats (represented by triglycerides) and easily cause cholesterol and other lipids to deposit on the vascular intima. Those over 40 with obesity should appropriately control food intake, maintain weight without excessive increase, and use a low-fat, low-cholesterol diet. Those already diagnosed with coronary heart disease, especially patients with elevated blood cholesterol, need to pay more attention to proper diet control. Other heart disease patients should similarly avoid excessive obesity to increase heart burden, strictly prohibit overeating and drinking, strive for a light diet, not eat too much, and eat more vegetables, fruits, beans and other foods.

5. Smoking and alcohol can cause increased heart rate, vasoconstriction, myocardial ischemia, hypoxia and arrhythmia, so heart disease patients should quit smoking and alcohol.

## 21. What should individuals with hypertension pay attention to when practicing Tai Chi Chuan?

The causes of hypertension are not yet fully understood, but it is generally believed to be due to dysfunction of the cerebral cortex. Intense, prolonged, and repeated external environmental stimuli acting on the cerebral cortex can cause mental tension and emotional excitement, leading to dysfunction of the cerebral cortex. This disrupts the mutual regulation and balance between the cortex and subcortical centers, causing dysfunction (tendency towards excitation) of the subcortical vasomotor center, resulting in the contraction of small arteries throughout the body and thus raising blood pressure.

If this state persists, it can cause the renal tissue to produce a substance called renin due to reduced blood supply. Renin interacts with another substance in the blood (angiotensinogen) to produce angiotensin, which has a constricting effect on small arteries throughout the body, further solidifying the already elevated blood pressure. Over time, this can lead to arteriosclerosis of small arteries and a series of other changes within the body, causing blood pressure to change from temporary or fluctuating elevation to stubborn and stable elevation.

However, not everyone exposed to adverse external stimuli will develop hypertension. This is related to individual constitution, nerve type, and genetic factors. The lack of proper training and exercise of the nervous system often causes abnormal reactions to certain stimuli. Tai Chi is one of the effective means of training and exercising the nervous system. Practice has shown that Tai Chi is effective not only in the prevention and treatment of hypertension but also in the prevention and treatment of hypotension. This indicates that Tai Chi can regulate blood pressure: it can raise low blood pressure and lower high blood pressure. The Sports Medicine Research Institute of Beijing Medical College found that the average blood pressure of elderly people who regularly practice Tai Chi is 101/80-8 mmHg, while that of the control group of elderly people who do not practice Tai Chi is 201:0/82:1 mmHg. The arteriosclerosis rate is

39.5% in the Tai Chi group, compared to 46.4% in the general elderly population. The Medical Sports Room of Huashan Hospital, Shanghai First Medical College, investigated 80 elderly people aged 50-79 who have been practicing Tai Chi for an average of 25 years, and compared them with 141 elderly people of the same age who do not practice Tai Chi. They found that the incidence of hypertension in the Tai Chi group is less than half that of the general elderly population. Research and practice in many places across the country now prove that long-term Tai Chi practice can lower or normalize blood pressure in hypertension patients, indicating that Tai Chi has a certain effect on the prevention and treatment of hypertension.

Some people do not achieve significant blood pressure-lowering effects due to improper Tai Chi practice methods. Hypertension patients should pay special attention to extreme relaxation of movements and extreme mental calmness during Tai Chi practice. This has a good relieving effect on pathological tension, emotional excitability, nerve sensitivity, tremors, and small artery contraction or vasospasm in hypertension patients, and is also an effective measure to reduce serum lipids and cholesterol. Additionally, one should achieve "upper body relaxed, lower body solid." Specifically, this means relaxing the shoulders, waist, chest, abdomen, and arms while shifting the tension point to the feet. This can stabilize the lower body, avoiding a top-heavy feeling, and has a certain effect on preventing cerebrovascular accidents.

Experiments have shown that sustained mental labor and mental tension can cause abnormal fat metabolism, increasing serum lipids and cholesterol. Therefore, one should reasonably arrange their life, study, work, and rest, and try to avoid factors that adversely affect the central nervous system, such as smoking, alcohol, and emotional tension. People over 40 should moderately limit foods high in cholesterol (such as animal fats and egg yolks) and should correctly approach illness, cultivating a revolutionary optimistic spirit. As everyone knows, hypertension mainly manifests as small artery contraction, and pleasant emotions can just cause small artery dilation. During treatment, blood pressure tends to fluctuate. Fighting chronic diseases is often not smooth sailing, and one must be mentally prepared for this, ready to face several relapses before finally overcoming the disease. For some more stubborn cases of hypertension, in addition to practicing Tai Chi, other comprehensive treatment measures should also be taken.

## 22. Why is Tai Chi Chuan effective in preventing and treating flat feet?

Flat feet, also known as fallen arches, can be congenital or acquired. Congenital flat feet may not always present symptoms, whereas acquired flat feet often result from prolonged weight-bearing activities or weakening of the body post-illness, leading to relaxed medial and deep lateral ligaments and reduced strength in the lower limb support muscles. This inability to withstand body weight pressure causes the normal arch, which does not touch the ground, to collapse, impacting bodily functions.

The active prevention and correction of flat feet involve rigorous exercise of the foot's ligaments and muscles, and Tai Chi Chuan is particularly focused on foot exercises. The full sequence of Tai Chi movements not only includes foot-focused techniques such as kicking, stepping, and swinging but also incorporates detailed and complex foot movements throughout each form. These include alternating the weight between the feet, advancing and retreating, toe pointing inwards and outwards, elevating and lowering, as well as left and right rotations of the heel and sole. Such movements significantly enhance the elasticity of the foot muscles and ligaments and maintain joint flexibility.

To prevent and correct flat feet during Tai Chi practice, it is essential to clearly differentiate between the weighted (solid) and unweighted (empty) stances, adapt the body's movements to the steps, and walk as softly as a cat. Some practitioners aptly point out that during fixed postures, the toes and heels should be firmly grounded, and the Yongquan point (located on the sole) should remain relaxed. Particularly, the toes of the foot bearing the body's weight should grip the ground as if grasping an object, while the entire sole should adhere to the ground as if using a suction cup. Then, with the shifting of weight, the toes should be gently relaxed. This rhythmic tightening and loosening activity provides thorough exercise to the entire foot's muscles and ligaments. With prolonged practice, the arches in most individuals will strengthen and become more resilient, leading to lighter and more agile movements. Over time, the inner side of the foot sole in individuals with flat feet can gradually regain its arch, effectively eliminating the condition. Even if the physical shape of the flat feet does not fully recover, symptoms like pain in the soles, calves, or back often lessen or disappear.

## 23. What should arthritis patients consider when practicing Tai Chi Chuan?

Arthritis generally includes common types such as rheumatoid arthritis, traumatic arthritis, infectious (gonococcal, undulant fever, dysenteric, tuberculous) arthritis, and arthritis of unknown etiology.

When joints are inactive for long periods, the surrounding muscles, joint capsules, and ligaments atrophy, and even joint cartilage may become uneven or be replaced by connective tissue. Traditional Chinese Medicine believes: "Pain leads to obstruction, obstruction leads to pain." Tai Chi, with its gentle movements and emphasis on muscle relaxation, helps alleviate muscle spasms, improves blood supply to muscles, and enhances metabolism in connected diseased tissues. There are many causes of pain in arthritis, one of the main common reasons being poor blood circulation, which stimulates nerve endings in various tissues or disrupts their nutritional metabolism. Appropriate exercise can improve the nutritional state of tissues surrounding the joints, reducing or eliminating adverse stimulation of nerve endings, thus relatively improving pain. However, the more pronounced the pain and joint deformity, the more attention should be paid to gentle and relaxed movements, gradually increasing the range of motion. Tuberculous arthritis is divided into allergic and metastatic types; the former can be exercised like general arthritis, while the latter is not suitable for Tai Chi practice. Arthritis patients practicing Tai Chi should also note the following points:

1. Progress should be gradual, with exercise intensity increasing from small to large, and the range of motion of affected joints should also gradually increase, limited to the point where joints do not show redness, swelling, or burning pain. Muscle soreness after exercise is normal; a slight increase in original pain at the beginning of the exercise regimen should not be feared, and one should persist with the exercise. However, each exercise session should not overburden the affected joints to avoid acute recurrence.

2. During sudden weather changes, such as cold or strong winds, timely attention should be paid to keeping warm to prevent joints from getting cold or catching a cold.

3. During acute flare-ups of arthritis, rest is necessary, and Tai Chi practice should be avoided. Consume foods rich in various vitamins, calcium, and phosphorus to increase resistance.

## 24. Is there any benefit for manual laborers in practicing Tai Chi Chuan?

Tai Chi Chuan is suitable for people of all ages, physical conditions, and genders. However, is it appropriate and necessary for those engaged in manual labor? As we know, each type of manual labor has its own operational characteristics, typically involving continuous localized physical activities. This often results in certain muscle groups being overused while others remain relatively inactive, preventing comprehensive physical development. For example, activities like planting, weeding, and harvesting primarily stress the lower back and arms, while pulling carts and carrying loads mostly utilize the waist and legs. Due to the stationary nature of many types of work, repeated posture can lead to an uneven burden on the body and a lack of overall physical exercise. Over time, this can hinder balanced muscular development and even lead to deformities.

The benefits of integrating sports activities, especially Tai Chi Chuan, with manual labor are significant. Unlike manual labor, which often involves repetitive, localized tasks, sports activities typically engage various muscle groups across the body. Regular participation in sports can exercise the muscles, internal organs, and the nervous system, leading to more agile movements and increased strength during labor.

After a day of strenuous activity, engaging in sports might seem counterintuitive—might it not lead to increased fatigue? However, there are various forms of rest. Lying down is one method, but performing light activities to mobilize the body and relieve fatigue in overused muscles and organs is also effective. In everyday life, for instance, after prolonged bending, standing up and stretching can alleviate discomfort. Similarly, appropriate physical activities after labor can help eliminate fatigue and invigorate the spirit. This is known as active rest. Of course, the intensity should be appropriate; after a particularly exhausting workday, engaging in strenuous exercise is not advisable. Light activities like walking or practicing Tai Chi Chuan are sufficient.

Tai Chi Chuan, which emphasizes relaxation, is particularly beneficial after physical labor. It enables comprehensive, relaxed bodily movements that can significantly aid in fatigue recovery. The holistic movements required in Tai Chi Chuan, which engage both internal and external aspects of the body, not only promote overall physical development but also play an active role in preventing and correcting certain occupational diseases.

Evidence shows that many older individuals, including peasants and workers in their sixties and seventies, have maintained robust health and continued full-day labor participation due to their long-term commitment to practicing Tai Chi Chuan. This demonstrates that Tai Chi Chuan is not only suitable but beneficial for manual laborers, enhancing their physical capabilities and overall well-being.

# 25. What are the benefits of practicing Tai Chi Chuan from a young age?

According to observations by the Qingdao Epidemic Prevention Station, practicing Tai Chi Chuan from a young age offers several benefits.

### Promotes Normal Development in Children and Adolescents:

Tai Chi Chuan is typically practiced in two ways: one involves slow, relaxed, and gentle movements suitable for the elderly and those with chronic diseases; the other combines slow and fast movements, both soft and strong, which is more suitable for children and adolescents. Tai Chi Chuan engages both internal and external aspects of the body, with every part in constant motion during practice. This full-body engagement, clear stepping patterns, steady yet agile movements, and deep, natural breathing contribute to enhancing the function of vital organs like the heart and lungs. It promotes blood circulation and metabolism throughout the body, increases flexibility and elasticity of joints, tendons, and muscles, and supports bone growth.

### Enhances Physical Qualities in Children and Adolescents:

Tai Chi Chuan incorporates a variety of movements in its basic skills, forms, and supplementary exercises, including bending, rising, twisting, jumping, leaping, and balancing. These movements demand different hand forms, footwork, body methods, and visual focus, thus developing flexibility, agility, endurance, speed, strength, and coordination in young practitioners.

### Helps in the Preservation and Promotion of Cultural Heritage:

Tai Chi Chuan is a valuable cultural heritage of China, born from the wisdom of the Chinese working people. It is not only a popular and highly encouraged form of exercise among the Chinese populace but also a sport and art form admired and embraced in many countries around the world. Many foreigners appreciate and desire to learn Tai Chi. Starting from a young age, practitioners can achieve a higher level of skill and have more favorable conditions for advancing in Tai Chi than those who start as adults.

In conclusion, practicing Tai Chi Chuan from a young age offers extensive health benefits, enhances physical capabilities, and provides a profound connection to an important aspect of cultural heritage. These benefits underscore the value of introducing Tai Chi Chuan early in life, facilitating not only physical development but also cultural appreciation and personal discipline.

# Chapter Three

## Tai Chi Chuan Push Hands, Implements, and Instruction

### 1. What is Push Hands and Sensing Energy?

Push hands, also known as joining hands, squeezing hands, striking hands, or connecting hands, is one of the methods used by ancient people to exercise the body or engage in close combat with enemies. Push hands is a two-person exercise using methods from Tai Chi such as ward-off, roll-back, press, push, pluck, split, elbow strike, and shoulder strike. In addition to the above methods, San Shou (free sparring) also includes kicking, striking, throwing, and grappling. It is a form of practical combat practice with resistance. Because push hands involves close contact between two people, those with infectious diseases such as tuberculosis or infectious hepatitis should consciously refrain from participating in this activity to avoid infecting others.

Push hands is a resistance exercise that can increase interest. It can also train "understanding energy", which means enhancing one's sensory abilities through push hands. After practicing push hands to a certain level, when an opponent's hand or body part touches one's own body, one can immediately perceive the source, path, and intensity of the opponent's energy, then adhere to or stick to the opponent's hand so it cannot easily escape. One can skillfully use the opponent's energy against them, gaining a completely advantageous position and using mechanical principles to send the opponent away. This is achieving "understanding energy", which is the martial significance of push hands. It must be emphasized that our purpose in practicing push hands today is to strengthen our physical condition, and we should implement the principle of "friendship first, competition second". Some people use push hands to deceive and do evil, which should be severely criticized and resisted. After understanding energy, push hands becomes increasingly refined. In other words, only after learning to understand energy will push hands progress quickly, achieve high effectiveness, and allow techniques to be applied freely. There are many methods and forms of push hands, with the following commonly used:

## Single joining hands:

Two people face each other, each stepping forward with the right (or left) foot, touching the back of the right (or left) wrist, and pushing back and forth.

## Single-hand horizontal circle push hands:

Each person joins one hand, making horizontal circular pushing and rubbing movements.

## Single-hand vertical circle push hands:

Each person joins one hand, making vertical circular pushing and rubbing movements.

## Single pressing push hands:

Two people each join one hand, making back and forth pressing wrist movements.

## Double joining hands:

Right hand and footwork same as single joining hands, but each person's left palm supports the opponent's elbow. Four arms join together forming a circle.

## Roll-back and push method:

When pushing hands, only perform roll-back and push movements.

## Roll-back and press method:

When pushing hands, only practice roll-back and press movements.

## Press wrist and push elbow method:

Four arms join together, making pressing wrist and pushing elbow movements.

## Four primary push hands:

When pushing hands, practice ward-off, roll-back, press, and push movements (divided into stationary and moving step versions).

## Four corner push hands (commonly called "big roll-back"):

When pushing hands, practice pluck, split, elbow strike, and shoulder strike movements. On the surface it looks like all roll-back movements, so it's also called "big roll-back".

## 2. What Does "Jin" Refer to in Tai Chi Chuan? How to Enhance "Internal Jin"?

The distinction between li (口) and jin (口) has long been a topic of debate among martial artists. Tai Chi advocates "using intent rather than force," but also emphasizes the use of jin, which can be confusing for beginners. In reality, jin and li are generally consistent; completing movements without the force of muscle contraction is impossible, and even maintaining posture requires muscle support. However, the jin required in Tai Chi is a flexible, concentrated, and freely applied elastic force developed through long-term practice (elastic force also varies in size, and those who are weak should not use larger elastic force). To develop this force, one must not only focus on practicing muscle tension and contraction strength but also on training sensitivity and quick reactions, while emphasizing the use of correct techniques to reasonably exert muscle strength. Therefore, it differs from the tense, rigid force of those who have not practiced Tai Chi or are not proficient in it. The "force" in "using intent rather than force" refers to avoiding tense, rigid, or excessive force.

When analyzing human posture and movement, one must consider the effects of external and internal forces and study the relationship between them. The main external force on the human body is gravity, which is the body weight due to Earth's attraction. Other external forces include support reaction force, friction, fluid force, and inertia. During push hands, one party's muscle force is also an external force to the other party. Tai Chi is a holistic exercise where bones and ligaments are the passive parts of the movement apparatus (levers), and muscle contraction is the active part (power). The internal force generated by muscle contraction is the "internal jin" in martial arts. Muscle contraction and relaxation, muscle tension, and length changes are all regulated by the central nervous system. Specific muscle groups participate in specific movements, and isolated muscle contraction does not occur. Moreover, as mentioned earlier, when a group of synergistic muscles contracts, the opposing muscle group (antagonistic muscles) must relax.

Beginners in Tai Chi often consume a lot of unnecessary energy because some muscles that are useless or even obstructive to completing the movements also participate in the work. As a result, unnecessary muscle tension and contraction cause rigidity in areas where force should not be applied, while the relaxation of antagonistic muscles in areas where force should be applied leads to partial cancellation of the force, making the entire movement tense and rigid. As one becomes more proficient in Tai Chi and push hands, unnecessary muscle tension can gradually be eliminated, and the ability to appropriately distribute muscle tension can be developed. This is why jin in push hands is much more powerful than rigid force (tense, stiff force) to the opponent.

Practicing Tai Chi forms and push hands can cultivate coordination in movements, which means training the central nervous system to send stimuli of specific frequency and intensity to specific muscle groups in a specific order. Therefore, the main goal in Tai Chi forms and push hands practice is to learn to adapt positive internal force (muscle work) to the reactive external force, quickly and accurately generating internal force through neural control to overcome, utilize, and counteract external force. Especially in push hands, the external force of each party constantly affects their internal force, causing corresponding internal force and, to some extent, determining the magnitude, direction, point of action, and duration of internal force. Similarly, internal force can also cause a series of external forces. For example, if the opponent attacks me with a pressing force, it is their internal force generated by muscle contraction; for me, this pressing force applied to my body is the external force from the opponent. If I respond with a pushing force, it is my internal force generated by muscle contraction, induced by the opponent's external force applied to my body; for the opponent, it is the external force I apply to them, induced by their internal force applied to me. If my internal force is greater, the external force I apply to the opponent will be greater, and if the opponent's internal force remains unchanged, they will be pushed out; if the opponent can increase their internal force to counteract my external force, both forces will balance and stalemate; if the opponent can further increase their internal force to overcome and exceed my external force, I will be pressed out. If the opponent uses my external force to change tactics, such as dodging, my pushing force will miss; for me, the internal force generated by my muscle contraction becomes an external force (inertia) acting on myself, causing me to fall in the direction of the pushing force. If I can quickly generate internal force in the opposite direction through muscle contraction to counteract this external force (inertia), I can stabilize myself. Thus, internal and external forces are mutually generated, influenced, and transformed between both parties, within the body, and between the body and the external environment.

How can one quickly enhance internal jin (internal force) or muscle elastic force? Using intent to direct movements and emphasizing coordination and relaxation is an excellent method. Muscle contraction is controlled by the central nervous system; the same muscle, when receiving high-frequency, high-intensity "commands" from the central nervous system, will have more muscle fibers contracting simultaneously, resulting in stronger contraction force. Additionally, coordination training ensures that muscle groups work together harmoniously, with antagonistic muscles relaxing appropriately to avoid cancellation, allowing the force to be effectively exerted. Furthermore, the increase in force depends on the extent of muscle stretch beforehand. Muscles that are already stretched (relaxed) before contraction can exhibit greater force during contraction. Therefore, emphasizing relaxation and naturalness will enhance muscle elastic force, making it more flexible and readily available. If physical strength, health, and age conditions permit, incorporating some obvious rigid force (without losing elasticity) during Tai Chi practice can also effectively increase internal jin. Regular push hands practice is also a primary means of enhancing internal jin.

## 3. What are Sticking, Adhering, Connecting, and Following? What Common Issues Arise in Push Hands?

Sticking, Adhering, Connecting, and Following are essential principles to observe during Push Hands. They entail maintaining an appropriate level of contact between one's arms and the opponent's arms, ensuring that no matter how actions may change, the contact does not break. Here's an explanation of these four principles:

## Sticking (Zhan):

This refers to initiating an upward lifting force. When joining hands with an opponent, one uses the opponent's resistance to lift their arm upwards, creating a tension in their upper body and a lightness below, possibly even lifting their heels off the ground. This aims to facilitate expelling the opponent. For beginners, understanding this force can be challenging; it's akin to bouncing a ball on a hard surface, where the force must be just right and elastic. Properly applied, sticking force resembles this bouncing action.

## Adhering (Nian):

Regardless of how the opponent changes their hand or body movements, one's arm never leaves the opponent's arm, as if gluing to them. This force, combined with sticking, is referred to as "sticking-adhering force."

## Connecting (Lian):

In Push Hands, one must remain continuously connected with the opponent, consciously linking one's force with theirs to gain a deeper understanding of their strength.

## Following (Sui):

This involves matching the opponent's movements in speed and direction, advancing and retreating in sync. As long as contact is maintained, one should not let the opponent escape regardless of their efforts, and this persistence is key to gaining the upper hand.

During the initial stages of learning Push Hands, beginners often struggle with sensing energy and commonly encounter problems of "losing touch" or "resisting." Losing touch refers to breaking contact with the opponent, while resisting is when one's force directly opposes the opponent's force. To properly execute sticking, adhering, connecting, and following, and to avoid these errors, one should engage with intent rather than brute force. This requires moving not based on subjective intentions but in response to the objective conditions of the opponent's movements, a concept in Tai Chi known as "abandoning oneself to follow the other." This principle applies not only to the hands but also to body positioning and footwork. All movements should be coordinated, neither leading nor lagging, flexible in response to the opponent's actions, thus avoiding disconnection, resistance, overextending, or counteracting. The ultimate goal is to respond adaptively to the opponent: retreating as they advance, advancing as they retreat, following when they rise, and relaxing when they sink. By using visual observation and more importantly, sensory perceptions such as touch and pressure, one can detect changes in the opponent's force direction and magnitude. This allows one to guide the opponent into a compromised position where their movements become passive. At such a moment, when the opponent is least capable of responding flexibly, one can expel them or seize them using a capturing force.

## 4. What is the Dialectical Relationship Between Curved and Straight Forces in Tai Chi Chuan Push Hands?

As discussed earlier, Tai Chi Chuan movements typically involve circular, arc-shaped, or spiral motions. Does this mean there is no straight force in Tai Chi Chuan? Indeed, there is straight force, and the curved and straight forces are interdependent and transform into each other. The principle of "seeking straightness within curvature and accumulating before releasing" encapsulates this dialectical relationship. Consider the example of drawing a bow and shooting an arrow: without the curved accumulation of energy in the bow, the arrow could not shoot straight. Of course, straightness is relative, not absolute.

In Tai Chi Chuan Push Hands, practitioners often stabilize their posture during the curved accumulation phase. If one can pinpoint the opponent's compromised posture, and if the point, direction, and timing of contact are correctly chosen, a straight force can be effectively released. For instance, if you strike a spherical ball with a straight rod aimed directly at its center of gravity, the ball will travel far. However, if the point of contact or direction is off, the ball might move and rotate but will not go far.

The direction in which straight force is applied during Push Hands depends on specific circumstances. For example, if the opponent is in a right bow stance with the right foot forward and the left foot back, applying force perpendicular to the line connecting their feet can easily expel them. Additionally, straight forces often incorporate spiral movements.

Conversely, when an opponent applies a straight force, using a curved or lateral force can neutralize it. Employing the "flashing and fighting" body method in combination can also be crucial, as it allows a smaller force to overcome a larger one, shifting from a passive to an active state. Thus, the point of application on the arms during movements constantly changes. Once the effect of one point is surpassed, another point is used, creating a series of curves and straight lines. Everywhere there is sticking force, and everywhere there is releasing force.

In the continuous transformation of maintaining and countering positions, any point along the circular path can potentially become a straight line from which force is projected. If there is only circular force without straight force, one can only neutralize but not release force. If there is only straight force without circular force, any attempt to neutralize will fail, leaving one vulnerable to an opponent's attack. Therefore, curved and straight forces are opposites that complement each other, mutually dependent and constraining.

## 5. Why is it said that "to retreat is to prepare to advance" in Push Hands?

The approach of never allowing even a slight retreat, favoring only hard, aggressive forward movements without blocking or parrying, only works when there is a significant disparity in strength and technical superiority. However, this approach often fails in Push Hands and does not achieve the goals of fitness and health. When the strength and skill levels are similar, especially when the weaker faces the stronger, those who recklessly advance without choosing the right moment often face setbacks in practice. Chairman Mao insightfully noted: "It is well known that when two boxers compete, the smarter boxer often takes a step back, letting the opponent unleash their full capability aggressively, which often results in the aggressor being defeated" (from "Problems of Strategy in China's Revolutionary War," Selected Works of Mao Zedong, p. 187). This vividly points out the dialectical relationship between retreating and advancing.

In Push Hands, where the weaker aims to overcome the stronger, it's crucial not to advance without ever retreating. However, retreating should not be misunderstood as merely a passive or escapist action. Nor should it be misconstrued as the old boxing theories often preach, such as "accepting what comes" or "winning without fighting". This requires critical examination. In reality, the purpose of retreating is to facilitate a more effective attack or counter-attack, which is key to victory. By retreating, one can "lead into emptiness," causing the opponent's forceful attack to miss, gather one's own strength during the retreat, or lead the opponent into a disadvantageous position, creating an opportunity for their error. The timing of the counter-attack depends on specific circumstances; it is effective when the opponent's weaknesses or mistakes are observed, when their excessive force compromises their stability and balance, or when their attack results in an unstable position, all of which are opportune moments to initiate a counter-attack. Additionally, techniques such as retreating while launching an attack (using pulling force or a large pulling step to expel the opponent) can also be employed.

Retreating should not be narrowly understood as merely moving backward with footwork. Even if the feet do not move, withdrawing the hands to draw the opponent in is also a form of retreat. Particularly in conjunction with body twisting and dodging maneuvers, where the left hand retreats allowing the right hand to advance simultaneously, and the retreating left hand also restrains the opponent. This is what is meant by "the returning hand hooks or doesn't return emptily," aimed at manipulating the opponent to facilitate a counter-attack and victory. It should be noted that retreating once does not always create an opportunity for a successful attack; sometimes, multiple cycles of advancing and retreating are necessary to secure victory.

## 6. What does "Gold Shoulders, Silver Chest, Tin Wax Belly" mean in Push Hands?

"Gold Shoulders, Silver Chest, Tin Wax Belly" describes the effectiveness of targeting specific body parts during Push Hands to cause an opponent to rotate, shift position, or fall. According to this saying, attacking the shoulders (gold) is most effective, the chest (silver) is less so, and the belly (tin wax) is the least effective. This classification is based on practical experience from practitioners and aligns with principles of mechanics.

Consider dragging two circular disks in the same direction with equal force. If the force on one disk is applied through the center point, this force will only move the disk in the direction of the force. However, if the force on the other disk is applied not through the center but at the edge, this will cause the disk to both move and rotate. Thus, even with equal force magnitude and direction, the different points of application produce different effects.

Applying this to Push Hands, if an opponent pushes my left shoulder with their right hand, and I rotate my torso to the left without stepping (thus allowing their force to continue unimpeded), while simultaneously pushing their left shoulder with my right hand, it is easier to make the

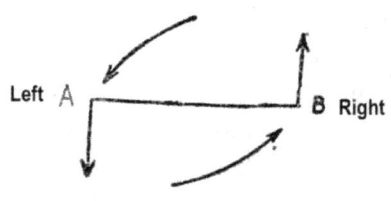

*Illustration 11*

opponent's body rotate. This technique is shown in Illustration 11. This is known as "left draw-right advance" or "left dodge-right advance," and similarly, "right draw-left advance" or "right dodge-left advance" can also be executed. If executed well, this can also transfer the opponent's force through my shoulder and spine to affect their body.

If instead of the shoulder, I push on the opponent's front chest, the rotational effect on their body is significantly reduced. If I push the opponent's left shoulder and they feel unstable, causing them to quickly withdraw their right hand, the pulling force they generate affects their right shoulder. At this moment, my right hand still exerts forward pressure on their left shoulder. Consequently, the opponent is subjected to two parallel forces in the same direction, and the resultant force (the combination of forces) is greater, compelling them to step back or even fall, as illustrated in Illustration 12.

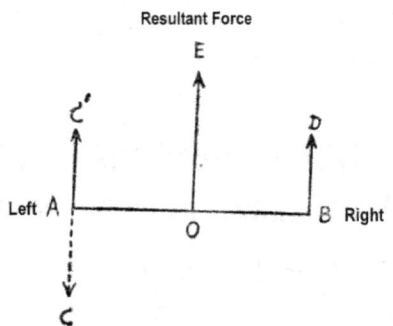

*Illustration 12*

## 7. Why is the Upward Pressing Force More Effective in Pushing the Opponent?

Applying horizontal force directly against an opponent's chest, if the opponent resists strongly, a stalemate occurs if both parties exert equal force. If the opponent's force is lesser, they are pushed back; if mine is lesser, I am pushed back. However, if the forces are not drastically different and my force is somewhat weaker, I can still gain advantage by applying force with the base of my palm towards the opponent's upper back area, or by adding an upward friction force with my palm and fingers while pushing directly. This creates a composite force AD directed upwards and backwards, increasing the force felt by the opponent, lifting them slightly off their toes, and causing their body to lean backwards—all of

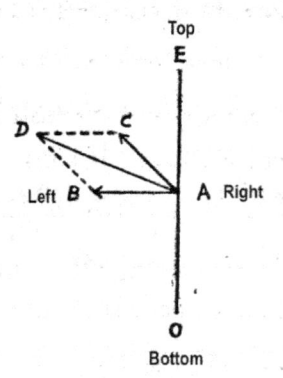

*Illustration 13*

which are disadvantageous for the opponent. Therefore, using upward pressing force (Warding Off) tends to be more effective in moving the opponent (illustrated in Illustration 13).

Conversely, when pushing towards the lower back area of the opponent, it is important to observe the direction of the support of the opponent's rear leg. For instance, if the opponent's right leg is supporting from behind, pushing directly towards the lower right back area can waste some force. According to the parallelogram law of forces, this force divides into two components: one component AC, which is canceled out by the reactive force from the supporting leg, leaving only the other component AB as the effective force moving the opponent's body (illustrated in Illustration 14).

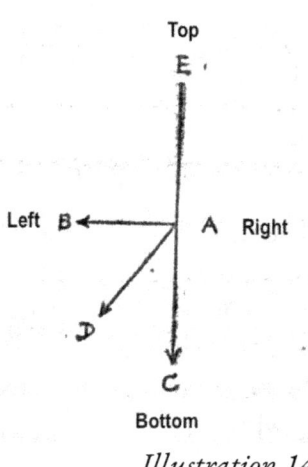

Illustration 14

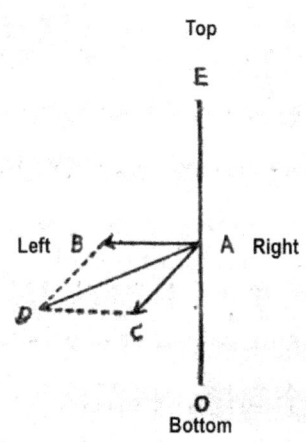

Illustration 15

Therefore, when pushing towards the opponent's lower back area, besides utilizing the downward force of the opponent's body sinking (to create a resultant force), it's also important to adjust the angle of application: if the right leg is behind, push slightly towards the lower left; if the left leg is behind, push towards the lower right. If the opponent still does not move, I can increase the force in the direction of AC (as shown in Illustration 15) to compel the opponent to resist upwards, at which point I immediately add upward force (as shown in Illustration 13). This is in line with the martial concept of "lifting to disrupt." If the opponent sinks down in response and my force does not lift them, I can also immediately withdraw the upward force, causing the opponent to lose their grounding. If the opponent lacks the technique to step and adjust quickly, or cannot move their feet swiftly enough to regain balance, their body will lean forward and become unstable. At this moment, by applying additional force, I can often achieve the desired effect; or if the opponent struggles to recover from leaning forward by straining backwards, I continue using the upward pressing force, which often proves effective.

## 8. How can you stand firm when pushing hands?

The stability of an object is related to its weight, height, and base area. An object of the same weight is more stable if it is shorter and has a larger base area; conversely, if it is taller with a smaller base, it tends to be less stable. This principle demonstrates that an object is more stable when it has a low center of gravity and a large supporting base; inversely, a high center of gravity and a small support base result in instability.

When standing in Push Hands, stability depends on the stance adopted, such as the height of the center of gravity, the size of the support base, the position of the center of gravity's vertical line within the base, and the muscle activity required to maintain this posture. The human body's center of gravity when upright is approximately between the first and fifth sacral vertebrae; some also believe it's about 2.5 cm below the navel, which may vary with body type and gender. During Push Hands, the center of gravity is generally kept low.

The supporting base when standing is formed by the area of the soles and the space between the feet. If the feet are close together and the stance is high, the body's center of gravity is higher, making the center of gravity's vertical line close to the edge of the support base and less stable. Conversely, a wider stance with a lower position, and the Qi sinking to the lower abdomen, lowers the center of gravity, making it more stable as the vertical line is further from the support base edge.

It must be acknowledged that even with a wide stance, stability in all directions is not guaranteed. For example, a stance wide side-to-side is unstable front-to-back; a stance wide front-to-back is unstable diagonally.

Also, a stance that is too wide and bent can impair flexibility and quick responsiveness in defense and offense and requires more energy.

To balance stability and flexibility in movement, adopting empty (xu bu) and bow (gong bu) stances in Push Hands is advantageous. Such stances, forming a triangular base, are relatively stable (shown in Illustration 16). With slightly bent knees and the upper body straight or slightly leaning forward, movement in a certain direction should start with the foot closer to that direction to widen the support base, followed by the other foot. During movement, the legs and feet should not be raised too high, as prolonging single-foot support raises the center of gravity and affects stability, hence the saying, "lifting one foot leaves the other half-empty." If initiating an attack, one might move the rear foot slightly forward first (old boxing texts refer to this as "inch step"), then slightly advance the front foot in the direction of the attack, allowing the full body's force to be utilized while maintaining balance.

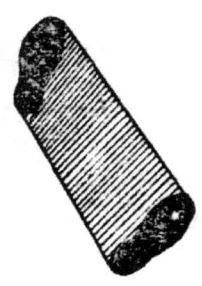

*Illustration 16*

In Push Hands, it is crucial to adeptly change the position of the lower limbs to compensate for any deficiencies in the support area. Adapting steps when losing balance helps maintain stability. Tai Chi Push Hands includes the concept of "double weight is ineffective, single weight leads to success," often seen in postures relying on one foot. Support on one foot offers a narrower base than two feet, appearing more likely to cause falling, yet it often leads to success. The key lies in the continuous adjustment of weight between the feet, adapting to the body's need for stability. If one foot becomes unstable, shifting the entire body weight to the other foot restores balance by constantly adapting the support base to shifts in the center of gravity. Additionally, using stepping to regain balance when losing it can also create instability or disadvantage for the opponent. For instance, if an opponent pulls me towards their diagonally rear side, I might step one foot between their feet and use a leaning technique to both regain my balance and disrupt theirs.

Furthermore, there's the technique of "sparrow hopping" when pushed to fall, which involves jumping back with both feet simultaneously to stabilize balance and prevent falling. The most commonly used method to maintain balance in Push Hands involves using the waist and hips as the axis for "transforming energy." When pushed by an opponent, rotating the waist and hips (coupled with the principle of "lifting energy"), and using techniques like rolling or plucking in the direction of the force towards the diagonal left or right not only maintains my balance but also causes the opponent to fall in the direction of the resultant force.

## 9. What does "Lightness Above, Solidity Below, Agility in the Middle" mean?

Based on the observations and research of predecessors, the body can be roughly divided into the upper body and lower body, with the place where the two parts meet being the waist. If further divided according to the integrity and function of the skeleton, the boundary between the upper and lower parts is between the fifth lumbar vertebra and the first sacral vertebra. But some people advocate dividing the upper body and lower body from the navel.

"Upper emptiness" refers to the upper body being empty and agile, "lower solidity" refers to the lower abdomen being heavy and solid. To achieve upper emptiness and lower solidity, simply put, it requires achieving: "emptiness, leading, top" and "empty, loose, drop." "Emptiness, leading, top" refers to the requirements for the head and neck posture, "empty, loose, drop" mainly refers to empty chest (broad chest), loose waist, and drooping buttocks. In this way, the body has an elastic force of being stretched up and down, making the upper body empty and agile but not floating, and the lower body heavy and solid but not rigid, thus resembling a hanging chain that is loose and flexible at every section, or like a floating buoy in fishing, swaying with the waves but always maintaining lightness above and heaviness below, also like a children's toy "roly-poly," with upper emptiness and lower solidity making it self-stabilizing and self-righting.

The requirement of upper emptiness and lower solidity in Tai Chi, especially relieving chest tension, is a very beneficial measure. For many people, especially those with neurasthenia, hypertension, etc., relieving mental tension and anxiety is very beneficial.

Expressions like "worried" and "anxious" indicate that some people often make their chest tense in daily life. There are also many situations in sports that make the chest tense, such as holding one's breath when exerting force. No matter the reason, chest tension will disrupt natural breathing, affecting the process of exhaling carbon dioxide and inhaling oxygen, and increasing chest pressure, affecting venous blood return to the heart, and even being detrimental to both large and small blood circulation. Some people practicing boxing make their jugular veins bulge, obviously because the blood circulation in the head and neck is obstructed due to chest tension. Therefore, it can be seen that relaxing the chest and leading with the top force is the key to upper emptiness.

How to achieve lower solidity? Mainly by achieving sinking shoulders and drooping elbows, containing the chest and pulling the back, and loosening the waist and drooping the buttocks. When pushing the arms forward, coordinating with natural exhalation, the tension in the chest can be sunk into the abdominal cavity with the counterforce of exhalation. While exhaling, containing the chest and pulling the back, sinking the shoulders and drooping the elbows, and gathering the lower qi, making the muscles of the shoulders, chest, and back naturally sink to the lower abdomen with exhalation, all help to sink the qi to the lower abdomen, also shifting the center of gravity downwards, thereby increasing the stability of the body and enhancing the sense of heaviness in the lower abdomen.

"Middle agility" refers to the requirement of being lively in the waist, which is handled very cleverly in Tai Chi, briefly mentioned in the answers about waist and hip posture, and further explored here.

The sacrum (i.e., the tailbone) is the cornerstone of the human body's pillar—the spine. However, the top of the sacrum is not level but tilted forward. This tilt angle is called the lumbosacral angle, represented by the angle between the top plane of the sacrum and the horizontal plane. The normal lumbosacral angle is 30-45 degrees, and some even reach 60 degrees. The upper body of a person "stands" on the sacrum through the fifth lumbar vertebra, just like "standing" on a steep slope (Figure 17). It is this relationship between the lumbar vertebra and the sacrum that makes the fifth lumbar vertebra always have a tendency to slide forward. The steeper the slope of the sacrum's forward tilt, the greater this sliding tendency. The impact of this tendency can be calculated using mechanical principles. Assuming a person's upper body weight is 100 jin (50 kilograms), and the lumbosacral angle is 30 degrees, then the forward sliding force is 50 jin (25 kilograms); if the lumbosacral angle is 40 degrees, it can reach 65 jin (32.5 kilograms); if the lumbosacral angle is 45 degrees, it can reach 70.7 jin (35.35 kilograms); if it is 50 degrees, it can reach 75 jin (37.5 kilograms); if it is 60 degrees, it can reach 86.6 jin (43.3 kilograms).

The increase in the lumbosacral angle not only increases the shear force (sliding tendency) of the lumbosacral joint but also affects the lumbar lordosis curve due to the increased slope of the sacrum. The larger the lumbosacral angle, the more the lumbar vertebrae protrude forward, the farther the lumbar vertebrae are from the center of gravity line, the greater the slope of each lumbar vertebra, the greater the shear force, and the harder it is to maintain balance. To maintain balance, the body inevitably makes certain tissues bear a greater burden, making it easy to fatigue or strain.

The sacrum and the iliac bones are closely connected, forming the pelvis. The drooping buttocks in Tai Chi actually involve a slight upward rotation of the pelvis, with the pubic symphysis slightly moving forward and upward, lowering the sacrum and reducing the lumbosacral angle. The lumbar lordosis curve also becomes smaller, which is called "straight waist" or "bow waist" (see the answers to questions about waist posture). Doing this is a crucial key to practicing Tai Chi well. Therefore, predecessors pointed out: "How can the body shape and waist top be absent, missing one is a waste of effort," emphasizing the importance of the head, neck, and lumbosacral. Only by properly gathering the buttocks (bending the hips and knees helps to gather the buttocks), reducing the hidden instability, can the spine "stand" on a smaller slope plane (reduced sacral slope), making the spine "stand" stably and move flexibly, making the middle (lumbosacral area) both solid and agile (Figure 18), and helping the qi and blood reach the toes of the solid leg, giving a sense of being rooted like a big tree. At the same time, because of the bending of the knees and hips, the legs contain a tendency for movement, making the solidity contain a sense of agility.

## 10. What Weapons are Included in the Tai Chi System?

In addition to the hand forms and Push Hands, the Tai Chi system includes various weapons, such as the Tai Chi sword, saber, and spear (staff). The requirements for practicing these weapons are fundamentally the same as for hand forms.

1. **In terms of movements**, the practice demands systematic coherence, uniform speed (though there are instances of quick force application), clear distinction between the substantial and the insubstantial, and natural breathing.

2. **In terms of body posture**, it is required to keep the head upright and centered, the coccyx vertically aligned, the chest contained and the back pulled up, with the shoulders sunk and the elbows drooping.

3. **Psychologically**, practitioners must focus intensely, keep their spirits contained, concentrate their thoughts, and use intent rather than brute strength.

Traditionally, Tai Chi Chuan did not include weapon forms; swords, sabers, and spears were developed later by adherents who applied the principles and characteristics of Tai Chi Chuan. Since the hand form is the foundation for weapon training, it is advisable for practitioners to first master the Tai Chi hand forms to establish a solid base before gradually learning the sword, saber, and spear techniques.

In terms of weapon form nomenclature, names that carry feudal superstitious connotations should be critically reformed. For example, in the Tai Chi thirteen spear techniques, the move "Child Worships Guanyin" has been changed to "Rest Step Withdraw Spear"; in Tai Chi sword, "Heavenly Horse Sailing Through the Sky" has been changed to "Empty Step Point Sword"; "Small Chief Star" has been changed to "Left Empty Step Swipe", and "Great Chief Star" has been changed to "Stand Alone Counter Thrust". Such reforms in naming are necessary not only to eliminate feudal remnants but also to make the names reflect the main contours of the movements, aiding in recall and memory.

# 11. What Challenges are Encountered in Learning Tai Chi Chuan?

Opinions on the difficulty of learning Tai Chi Chuan vary. Some people find it challenging, while others do not consider it difficult, believing that any obstacles can be overcome. As the great leader Chairman Mao taught us, "Nothing is difficult to the man who will try." In fact, years of teaching experience have shown that as long as one has a strong conviction to practice Tai Chi, carefully understands each movement and posture, and practices them repeatedly, anyone can learn Tai Chi Chuan. It's commonly said that "the first steps are the hardest." Initially, beginners may struggle with the unique style and characteristics of Tai Chi movements, finding them unfamiliar and uncomfortable. However, after a few days of practice and understanding the patterns of the movements, students tend to find them more approachable and gradually appreciate the lively and agile essence of this martial art. One of the key issues here is the method of teaching. For the more challenging aspects, the following teaching methods are generally adopted:

### Full-body Integration:

Each Tai Chi movement involves the entire body, often moving in arcs, circles, or spirals. Beginners may find it difficult to coordinate their left and right hands, or hands and feet simultaneously, especially in making circular, arc, or spiral movements without a basic athletic foundation. Teaching methods such as "start with straight then integrate circular movements," "set up the framework first," and "combine segmented and holistic approaches" can help students progress methodically and overcome these challenges.

### Weight Distribution and Leg Strength:

In everyday life, both legs equally support the body's weight. In Tai Chi Chuan, however, it is required to clearly distinguish between the solid and empty leg, with one leg often bent and bearing most or all of the body's weight. To address this challenge, many instructors begin by teaching footwork and stances, and by arranging for pole-standing exercises (stances) as part of the training.

In conclusion, instructors should tailor their teaching plans and methods to individual students, explain each posture or movement in detail, and use discussions to encourage students' active participation. Students, on the other hand, should establish a firm belief in practicing Tai Chi to strengthen the body for the revolution, ensuring they can effectively learn and master Tai Chi Chuan.

## 12. What teaching methods are commonly used in Tai Chi Chuan?

Tai Chi Chuan teaching methods vary depending on the students' level and the complexity of the movements. There are mainly two approaches: the holistic method and the segmented method.

### Holistic and Segmented Teaching Methods

The choice between holistic and segmented methods depends on the student's foundation and the simplicity or complexity of the movements. For students with a good foundation and simpler movements, the holistic method is appropriate. This method helps students understand the full scope of the movements and form a complete conceptual understanding, enabling them to master the actions in their entirety. This requires the movements to be coordinated and fluid. When students have a weaker foundation or the movements are complex, the segmented method is used to help them understand the details of the movements and accelerate their learning process. This might involve breaking down the movements into components such as footwork, hand techniques, or body movements, or dividing a sequence into several steps or movements. For example, "Grasping the Bird's Tail" can be explained in four parts: ward off, roll back, press, and push. However, the segmented method can disrupt the structure of the movements and affect their integrity. It also makes correcting ingrained habits more challenging. After using the segmented method, it is crucial to transition to the holistic method to ensure students master the complete movements.

## "Square First, Round Later" Teaching Method

The "Square First, Round Later" method is easy to grasp. It involves breaking down the circular movements of Tai Chi into linear, calisthenic-like actions. For example, the "Parting Wild Horse's Mane" movement from Simplified Tai Chi can be broken down into sitting back and lifting the leg, T-step holding the ball, and bow step parting the palms into three movements, with the footwork arranged in a zigzag pattern. Initially, students are only required to perform these movements without exerting force, simply focusing on the accuracy and structure of the positions. After mastering these movements, they should progress to more fluid and connected forms. This method is particularly suitable for students with poor coordination or athletic foundation. For movements requiring high coordination like "Roll Back" and "Cloud Hands," this method is also effective. In Tai Chi classes with diverse participants of varying skills without the possibility of specialized grouping, this method can achieve satisfactory results. However, for students with a solid foundation or in the later stages of learning sequences, it is advisable to continue using holistic and fluid teaching methods that integrate square and round movements.

The concepts of square (fang) and round (yuan), essentially, reflect the dialectic relationship between straight and curved. Attempts to explain this relationship using Tai Chi symbols, the eight trigrams, and other theories like the River Map and Luo Shu have only confused the issue further. In practice, numerous examples illustrate the productive interplay between square and round, such as in calligraphy, where students first practice standard script to establish a foundation with straight strokes before moving on to running or cursive script. In painting, artists often start with straight lines to draw geometric shapes for outlines. Once the contours are accurate, the overall image is captured, and the details pose little difficulty. Experience shows that the teaching method of starting with square then integrating round not only speeds up the mastery of routines but also ensures high-quality outcomes once the basic movements are grasped and effectively transformed into round movements. Students also report that this method is simple, clear, and adheres to a progressive learning pattern.

## 13. How to use Explanation and Demonstration in teaching Tai Chi Chuan?

In teaching Tai Chi Chuan, it is essential to adopt "inquisitive" and "discussion-based" methods rather than "instructive" ones, actively engaging students' initiative. For elderly, physically weak, or chronically ill individuals, it is beneficial to introduce examples of Tai Chi's effectiveness in treating chronic conditions and its preventive health benefits, helping them build a resolute determination to combat their illnesses. It should also be noted that experiencing muscle soreness in the legs and arms during the initial stages of training is a normal physiological response. For younger, stronger students, the health benefits of Tai Chi should be emphasized to dispel any misconceptions that Tai Chi is too slow or insufficiently vigorous.

When explaining, the language must be concise, easy to understand, vivid, and interesting, not only providing students with relevant knowledge but also guiding them to establish correct action concepts through thinking.

Therefore, to explain well, the teacher must make a plan in advance and pay attention to the following points:

## Focus on Key Points:

Avoid covering too much in one session. Use breaks or the last few minutes of class to address one or two key points with emphasis on their ideological significance.

## Use Mnemonics and Analogies:

Employ vivid language, such as mnemonics and metaphors, which can be highly effective. Many Tai Chi postures have names that vividly describe the actions, such as "Play the Lute," which visually resembles playing the instrument and leaves a lasting impression. Introducing actions like "Embrace the Ball" across various movements can significantly aid beginners in remembering and mastering the sequence of movements. For instance, "Part Wild Horse's Mane" consists of an embrace on the side and diagonal palm splits. Describing movements with vivid phrases like "step like a cat," "draw silk from cocoons," and "flow like drifting clouds" can deeply enhance the understanding of movement fluidity and continuity.

## Order of Explanation:

For more complex movements, it is generally effective to discuss footwork first, followed by upper limb and hand techniques. For example, in "Part Wild Horse's Mane," one might first explain the bow stance, then the footwork, and finally the upper limb actions like embracing and splitting the palms, culminating with the integration of upper and lower limbs and body methods.

## Analyze Defensive and Offensive Aspects:

Analyzing the martial applications of movements helps students grasp essential principles, making the actions more coordinated, complete, and precise. For example, "Part Wild Horse's Mane" can be broken down into warding, lifting, elbowing, and leaning techniques, which can be analyzed through paired practice to deepen understanding. However, it should be emphasized that the purpose of practicing Tai Chi is fitness for the revolution, and training solely for combat skills is discouraged.

Demonstrations allow students to directly understand the form, structure, and spirit of the movements. Accurate and graceful demonstrations can spark interest and facilitate understanding of the actions. Therefore, demonstrations should strive for correctness and practicality, avoiding showiness without substance.

Explanation and demonstration should be seamlessly integrated. You can explain first and then demonstrate, or vice versa, or even combine both simultaneously. Inviting students to perform while providing explanations can help quickly establish a comprehensive concept of the movement. Overall, both explanation and demonstration are critical in helping students quickly form a complete understanding of Tai Chi movements.

## 14. What Does It Mean to Practice or Frame the Framework? Is the Method of "Seeking Extension First, Then Compactness" Correct?

Practicing the sequence of Tai Chi movements in order is commonly referred to as practicing or framing the framework, also known as setting up the framework. The term "framework" here refers to the stance or posture used during practice.

The traditional boxing theory advocates "seeking extension first, then compactness," meaning that whether framing the framework or Push Hands, the postures should initially be practiced with larger, more expansive movements before transitioning to smaller, more compact ones to refine the technique. This approach is feasible for individuals who are physically robust. Larger movements involve greater range of motion in the waist and legs, while more compact movements involve a smaller range.

However, if the stance is too wide, it can hinder step transitions. If the stance is too low, it can cause the center of gravity to sink, which is not conducive to advancing, retreating, or changing between substantial and insubstantial stances. For example, in the bow stance, one leg is bent and the other is straight. The front leg should have the knee directly above the toes, which allows the waist to relax and facilitates rotational changes. Once proficiency is achieved, then one can practice making movements more compact. Some styles of boxing require movements to transition from large circles to smaller circles, and eventually, to almost no circles.

The principle of "seeking extension first" is not suitable for individuals with chronic illnesses or those who are physically weak. The larger the posture, the greater the amount of movement; the smaller the framework, the lesser the movement. Any Tai Chi sequence can be practiced in large, medium, or small frameworks. However, beginners must consider their physical capabilities and should not force themselves; they need to choose according to their strength. Elderly or chronically ill individuals should adopt smaller and higher stances. As their physical strength improves, they can freely choose to practice larger, medium, or smaller frameworks according to their preferences.

# Chapter Four

## Selection and Practice of Tai Chi Chuan

In order to broadly promote Tai Chi Chuan following the liberation, simplified versions were developed and various styles were systematized. This made the practice accessible and significantly beneficial in terms of fitness for the general populace. However, some individuals, especially workers and farmers, due to the nature of their labor and lifestyle, often find it challenging to complete a full set of Tai Chi Chuan routines or even to learn one fully. In response to this, we have compiled a selection of individual Tai Chi movements for practice.

Considering that many workers and farmers suffer from back and leg pains, we specifically chose movements that engage and enhance the flexibility of the waist, also increasing the range of motion in this area. Furthermore, to ensure a balanced development and exercise of the entire body, we adopted symmetric training methods and paid close attention to the coordination of movements with breathing.

This selective approach to practicing Tai Chi Chuan allows individuals to choose two or three movements to practice based on personal conditions and preferences, or to engage in the entire set. The exercises can be performed individually or in sequence, continuously, with no restrictions on the number of repetitions or speed, adapting the practice to personal, temporal, and environmental circumstances.

When compiling this selection, we endeavored to incorporate the strengths of various Tai Chi styles, taking into account the distinctive aspects of Tai Chi movements such as being empty or solid, opening or closing, rising or falling, and rotating or turning. In terms of posture, we focused on being 'empty' above, 'solid' below, and 'agile' in the middle. Our training methods emphasize being correct, slow, original, relaxed, even, and stable. The techniques incorporate pushing, pulling, squeezing, pressing, plucking, splitting, lifting, and leaning. Preliminary trials have demonstrated that beginners find it easy to learn and those with some foundation also see it as practicable. Due to its approachability, it facilitates widespread adoption and persistence, and the health and therapeutic effects are quickly evident.

For a comprehensive understanding of the physical requirements of each part of the body in Tai Chi Chuan, one can refer to the solutions provided for each topic in this book.

## 1. Preparatory Stance

Stand naturally with feet apart, about shoulder-width, toes pointing forward. Arms hang relaxed at your sides, hands resting on the outer thighs. Look straight ahead and pause briefly.

**Key Points:** Keep your head and neck upright, chin slightly retracted. Avoid deliberately puffing your chest or pulling in your abdomen. Focus your mind and relax all joints as much as possible (see Illustration 1).

## 2. Rising and Falling (Cupping and Pressing)

### Rising Cup:

Begin with hands cupped as if holding an object, slowly lift your arms straight forward without moving your legs, while inhaling (Illustration 2).

## Falling Press:

Turn hands so palms face downwards, bend knees to squat slowly while pressing down, exhaling simultaneously. The depth of the squat—full, half, or slight—depends on your physical condition (Illustration 3).

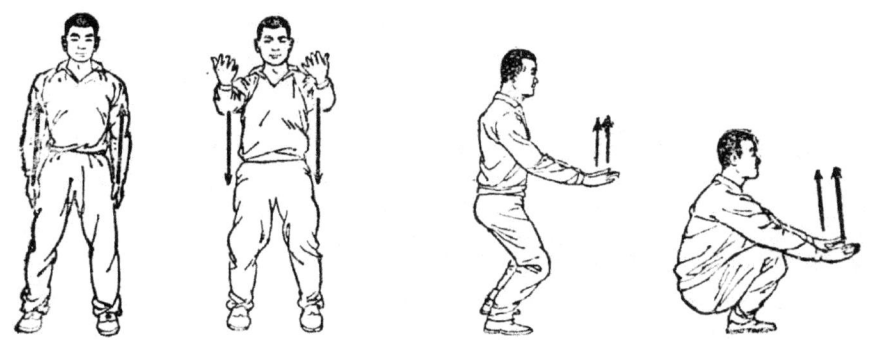

*Illustrations 1, 2, 3A and 3B*

Repeat these two steps several times.

**Key Points:** When rising, slightly push your head upward, and avoid sticking your buttocks out. Your posture should resemble a chain being pulled up and allowed to fall, with joints in the ankles, knees, and hips flexing sequentially. The upper body should maintain a straight posture like a chain.

# 3. Opening and Closing

## Bow Step Opening:

Step forward with your left foot, heel first making contact with the ground, then fully plant the foot while bending the left knee and keeping the right leg straight, forming a left bow stance. As you step and bend, move your hands to the sides and then together upward in front, palms facing inward, coordinating with a deep inhalation (Illustrations 4, 5).

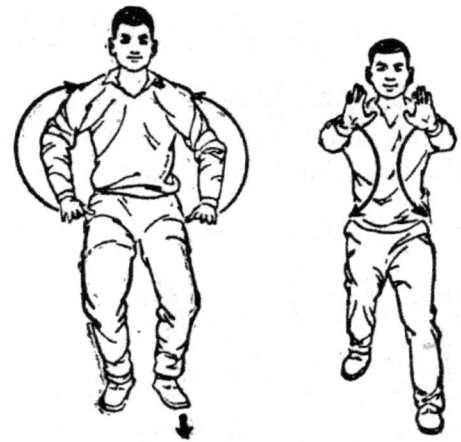

*Illustrations 4 & 5*

## Sitting Back Press:

Bend the right knee, sit back with your upper body, straighten the left leg, and raise the tip of your left foot (raising is optional), forming a left empty stance; at the same time, press both hands downward and backward, coordinating with a deep exhalation (Illustration 6).

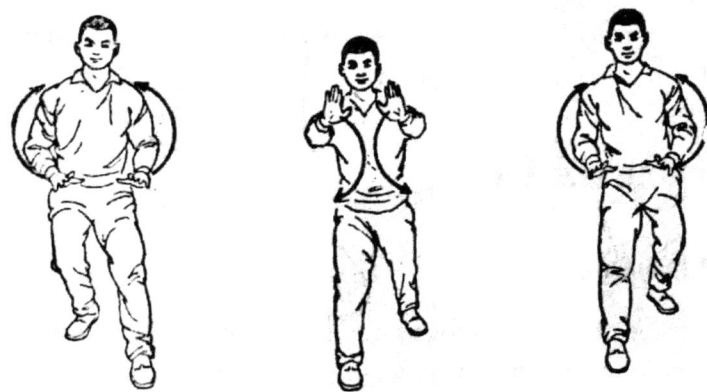

*Illustrations 6, 7 & 8*

Perform movements 4 and 5 so that your hands describe a diagonal circle from front to back and top to bottom. Repeat several times, and during the first movement (Illustration 5), step back to the original position with your left foot following your hands.

The movements 6 and 7 are the same as 4 and 5 but with opposite sides (Illustrations 7-8). After several repetitions, during movement 7 (Illustration 7), the right foot follows the hands back to the original position.

**Key Points:** Inhale softly; during exhalation, focus on dropping your shoulders and compressing inward.

## 4. Vertical Circular Elements

### Cupping and Squeezing:

Turn your body to the left (chest facing left), step out with your left foot forming a left bow stance; simultaneously, your left palm faces up and arcs forward and upward, while the right palm presses downward inside the left elbow, extending together with the left arm; your waist follows the arm's extension forward, palms facing each other at an angle, implying a squeezing motion (Illustrations 9, 10).

### Pressing:

urn the left palm downward and the right palm upward, bend the right knee, sit back with the upper body to form a left empty stance; both hands simultaneously draw an arc backward as if pulling a hoe during plowing, left hand to front left hip, right hand to front right hip (Illustrations 11, 12).

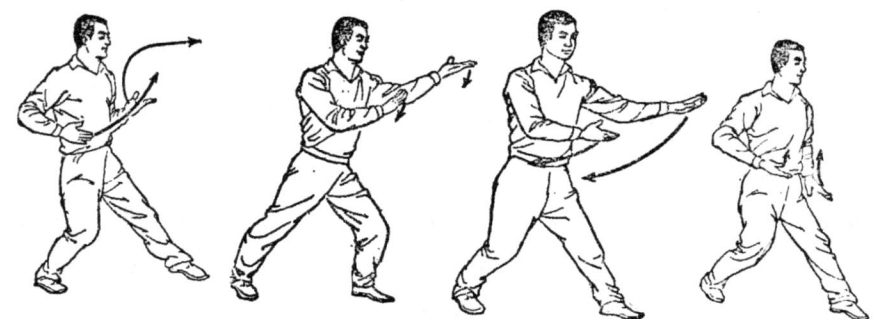

*Illustrations 9, 10, 11 & 12*

Repeat these movements several times.

Movements 13 and 14 are identical to 9 and 10 but in opposite directions (Illustrations 13-16), shifting from the second movement's direction (Illustration 12) toward the back.

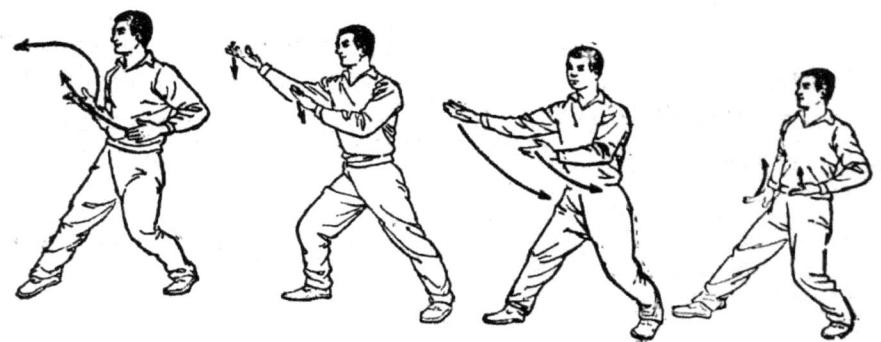

*Illustrations 13, 14, 15 & 16*

**Key Points:** Both palms must flip simultaneously, ensuring that "the palm exits as if from the mouth, and the returning hand goes back under the ribs." This ensures large and rounded movements, coordination between forward squeezing and backward sitting is essential.

**Simplified Practice Method:** Mimic the action of rowing with both hands, focusing on coordinating hand circles with waist and leg movements.

# 5. Horizontal Circular Elements in Tai Chi Chuan

For the specific movements and requirements for each part of the body, refer to this section.

## Bow Step Pushing and Squeezing:

Begin with the left knee bent in a left bow stance, simultaneously sweeping your left arm upward and to the left, palm facing upward and inward; right hand follows beneath the left elbow, pressing downward and outward with the palm facing downward (Illustration 17).

## Sitting Back and Hanging:

Slightly twist the waist to the left, as you bend the right knee and sit back, guide your left hand outward and back, hanging it above and outside the left shoulder, completing the movement in a left empty stance (with the left toe pointed up) as the hand reaches its final position (Illustration 18).

## Waist-Twisting Horizontal Movement:

Twist the waist to the right, both hands sweep horizontally to the right (Illustration 19).

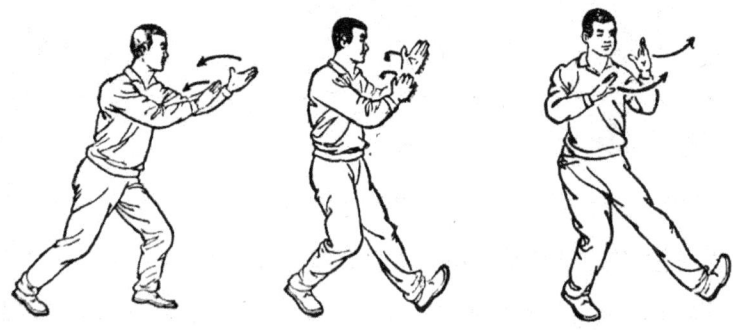

*Illustrations 17, 18 & 19*

## Bow Step Forward Press:

Twist the waist to the left, step firmly into a left bow stance with your left foot, both arms also turn with the waist, palms facing outward, pressing forward (Illustration 20).

Movements 21, 22, and 23 repeat the movements 17, 18, and 19 but in the opposite direction (Illustrations 21, 22, 23, 24).

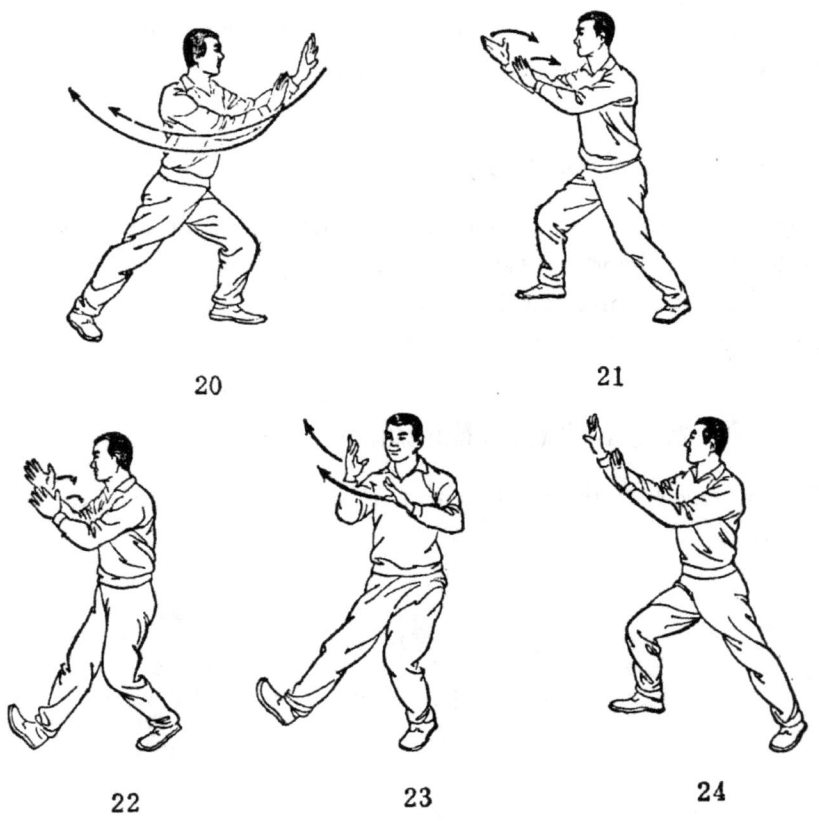

*Illustrations 20, 21, 22, 23 & 24*

Perform these alternating left and right movements several times to balance the elements.

**Key Points:** The arm's twisting and turning movements are driven by the waist, achieving what is described as "turning the axle through the spine and a rope around the waist," and "waist like a screw, legs like a drill."

**Simplified Practice Method:** Perform alternating left and right flag-waving movements. When waving to the left, the left hand is uppermost and the right hand lower, as if holding a flagpole, moving counterclockwise. When waving to the right, reverse the hands and move clockwise.

## 6. Diagonal Circular Elements (Parting the Wild Horse's Mane)

### Turning Body with Arms Crossed:

Turn right, shifting weight to the right, forming a right side bow stance, with right palm facing down and left palm up, arms crossed with the right arm on top (Illustration 25).

### Bow Step Parting Palms:

Turn to the left into a left bow stance, simultaneously left hand sweeps forward and upward in an arc, palm slanting up, level with the eyes, while the right hand sweeps back and to the right side, palm facing down, fingers pointing forward (Illustration 26).

Repeat movements 25 and 26 several times, each time the hands drawing a diagonal circle, with the left hand drawing a larger circle.

Movements 27 and 28 repeat the movements 25 and 26 but in reverse directions (Illustrations 27, 28).

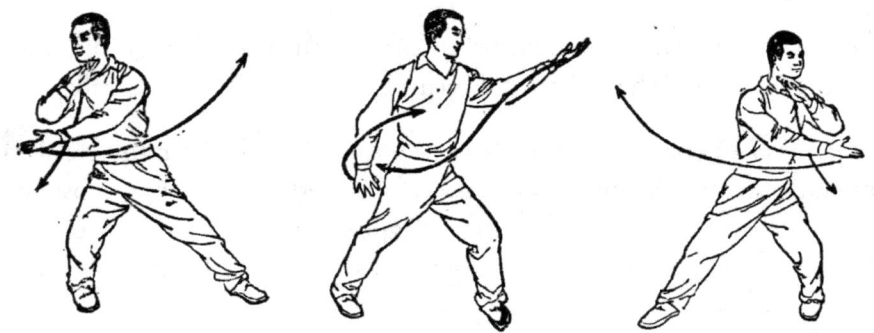

*Illustrations 25, 26 & 27*

**Key Points:** Arms are moved by the drive of the waist and spine, incorporating the four energies: plucking, toughness, elbowing, and leaning.

## 7. Brush Knee-Circling Step

### Right Hand Beard Stroking:

The right hand moves from outside across the chest (slightly left) downward in a beard-stroking motion, simultaneously turning the waist left, shifting body weight also to the left leg (Illustration 29).

### Left Hand Beard Stroking:

As the right hand strokes downward and outward, the left hand arcs from outside upward across the body (slightly right) in a downward beard-stroking motion, simultaneously shifting weight to the right and turning the waist right (Illustration 30).

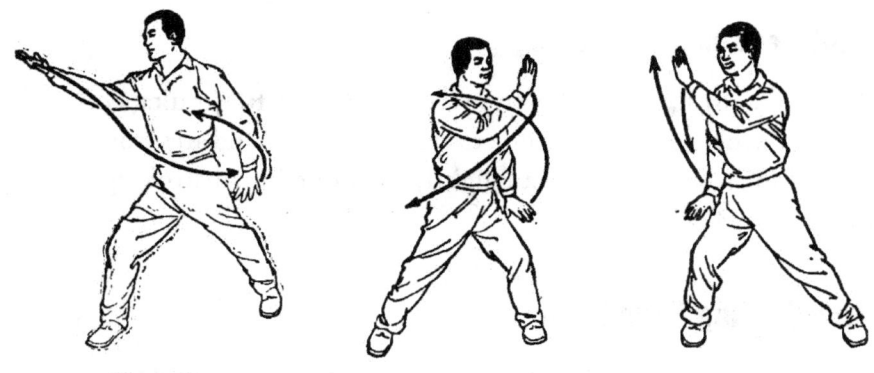

*Illustrations 28, 29 & 30*

## Knee-Circling Palm Push:

As the left hand circles the knee outward and down to the left, turn the body to the left, pushing the right hand forward from above past the ear, shifting weight onto the left leg forming a left bow stance (Illustrations 31, 32).

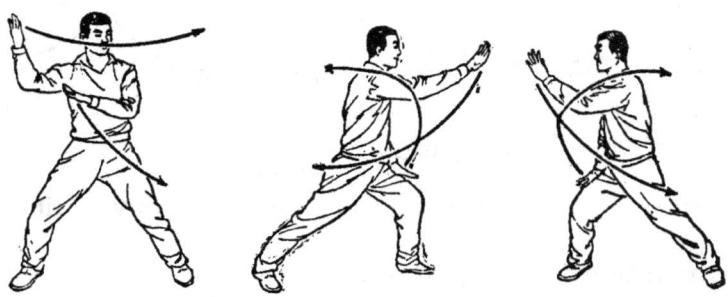

*Illustrations 31, 32, & 33*

## Left Hand Beard Stroking:

Turn the waist to the right, shifting weight to the right, simultaneously the right hand strokes downward and outward, the left hand arcs from outside upward to the front of the chest (slightly right) in a beard-stroking motion (Illustration 33).

## Right Hand Beard Stroking:

Turn the waist to the left, shifting weight to the left, simultaneously the left hand strokes downward and outward, the right hand arcs from outside upward in front of the chest (slightly left) in a beard-stroking motion (Illustration 34).

## Knee-Circling Palm Push:

Turn the body to the right forming a right bow stance, simultaneously the right hand circles the right knee, the left hand pushes forward from above past the ear (Illustrations 35, 36).

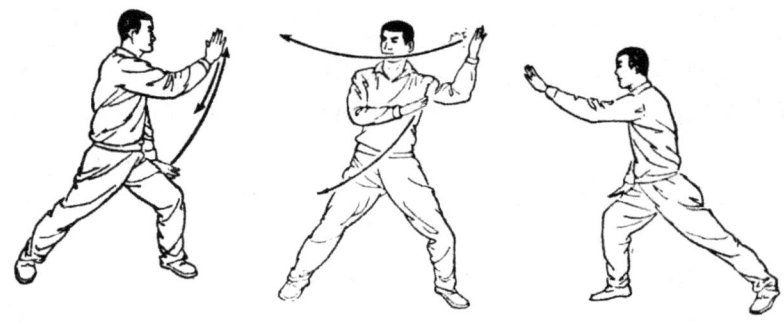

*Illustrations 34, 35 & 36*

Perform these left and right knee-circling palm pushes several times.

**Key Points:** Beard stroking must coordinate with the twisting of the waist, following the action, sinking the Qi to the lower abdomen.

**Simplified Practice Method:** With legs slightly bent and body relaxed, alternately perform beard stroking with both hands from top to bottom, driven by the movement of the waist and spine.

# 8. Cloudy Hands

### Left Cloudy Hands:

Shift your body to the left, adopting the left bow stance. Concurrently, your left hand, not rising above the eyebrows, sweeps across from above toward the left; simultaneously, the right hand, following the rotation of the torso, arcs from below (in front of the abdomen) towards the left shoulder (see Illustrations 37, 38).

### Right Cloudy Hands:

Rotate your body to the right, entering the right bow stance. At the same time, your right hand, also not exceeding eyebrow height, presses outward toward the right; the left hand, following the torso's rotation, traces an arc from below (in front of the abdomen) to the right shoulder (see Illustrations 39, 40).

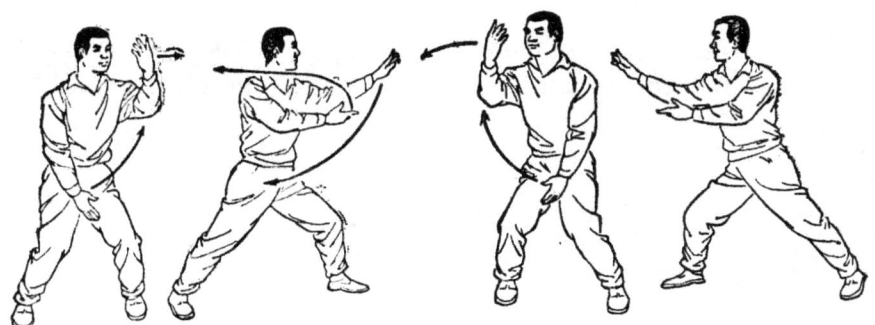

*Illustrations 37, 38, 39 & 40*

Repeat these rotations several times, alternating between left and right.

**Key Points:** Both hands must execute the lifting, warding off, turning, and pressing movements entirely driven by the movement of the lumbar spine. Engage the shoulders, twist the arms, and rotate the waist in a coordinated manner to achieve what is referred to as "turning the axle with the shoulder, waist as a twisting rope" and "waist like a screw, legs as drills."

# 9. Kicking

### Crouching and Embracing:

Draw your right foot beside your left, bending the knees into a full squat (a half-squat or slight squat is also permissible), while your arms embrace in front of you, left hand below, right hand above (see Illustration 41).

### Single Knee Raise:

tand on your right leg (knee slightly bent), lifting the left knee, with the toes naturally pointing downward, while your arms cross and embrace upward in a cross shape (see Illustration 42).

### Splitting Palm and Kicking:

Gently extend the left foot toward the left front, while both hands part from above towards the left front and right back, spreading out flat (see Illustration 43).

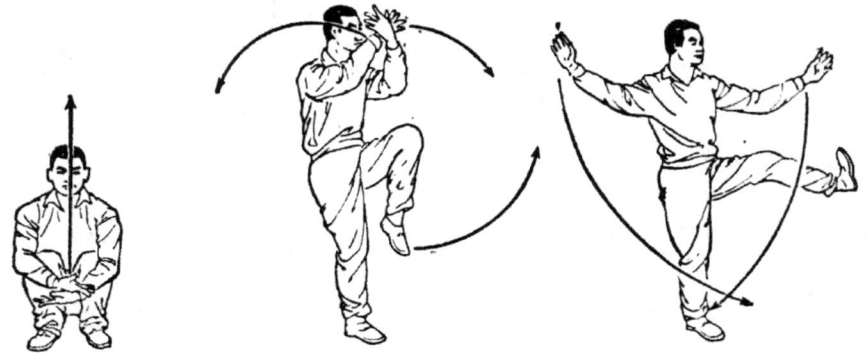

*Illustrations 41, 42 & 43*

Repeat the actions of 44, 45, 46 as the same for 41, 42, 43, but in the opposite direction (see Illustrations 44, 45, 46).

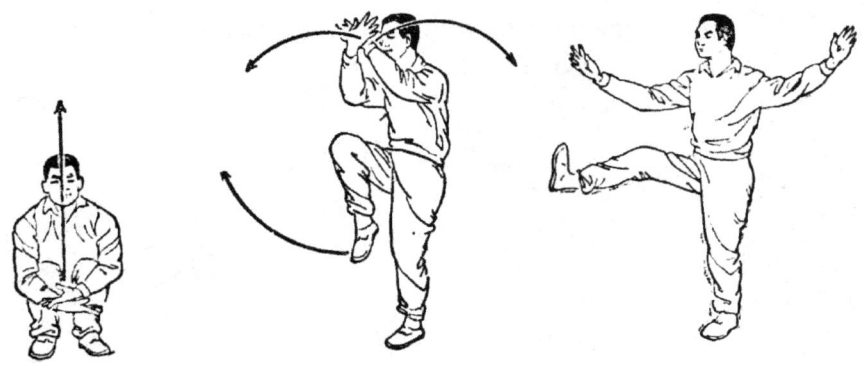

*Illustrations 44, 45 & 46*

Thus, one should alternately press down with each foot several times, shifting smoothly from left to right.

**Key Points:** Achieve lightness above and solidity below, ensuring coordination between the upper and lower body. The standing leg should be slightly bent for stability; the kicking foot must exert force through the heel with the toes pointing upwards.

# 10. One Leg Standing

## Stand on Right Leg:

Lift the left knee, entering the right stand-alone posture (right knee slightly bent), while the left hand moves from below upward in front of the body, palm facing up, and the right hand placed beside the right hip, palm facing down, fingers pointing forward (see Illustration 47).

## Stand on Left Leg:

Return the left foot to the original position, lifting the right knee, entering the left stand-alone posture, with the right hand moving from below upward in front of the body, and the left hand falling from above to beside the left hip (see Illustration 48).

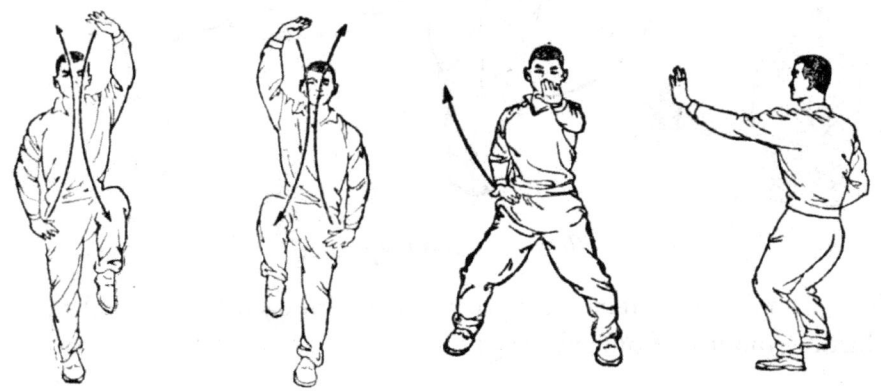

*Illustrations 47, 48, 49A & 49B*

**Key Points:** The standing leg's knee should be slightly bent, ensuring stability. The upper hand supports upward, while the lower hand presses downward simultaneously.

# 11. Horse Stance with Palm Push

## Horse Stance Palm Push:

Step the right foot approximately three feet to the right, squatting into a horse stance, while the left hand pushes from below upward in front of the body, and the right hand draws back to the waist, palm facing up (see Illustration 49).

## Waist-Turning Palm Support:

Twist the waist to the right, extending the right hand backward (palm still facing up), while the left hand flips with the palm facing up, slightly reaching forward as it flips. During this, gaze at the right hand (see Illustration 50).

## Palm Push:

Slightly twist the waist to the left, driving the right hand from beside the ear forward (palm facing forward), while the left hand withdraws back to the waist, palm facing up (see Illustrations 51, 52).

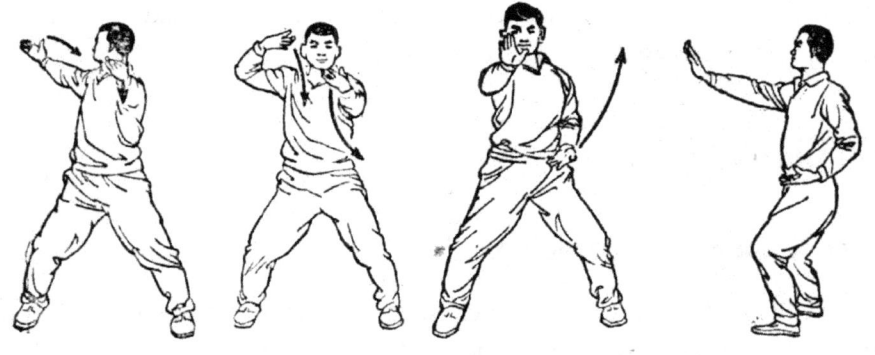

*Illustrations 50, 51, 52A & 52B*

## Waist Turning and Palm Upholding:

This movement mirrors the second action, with the distinction of being performed in the opposite direction (refer to Illustration 53).

## Pushing Palm:

This action replicates the third movement, but is executed with the opposite sides of the body (refer to Illustrations 54 and 49).

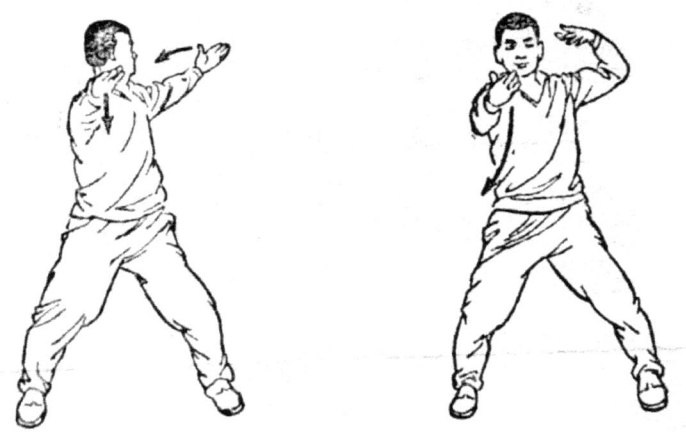

*Illustrations 53 & 54*

**Key Points:** Keep the waist active and the shoulders relaxed. The spine, acting as an axis, drives the arm movements.

# 12. Closing Form

## Arm Circling and Embracing:

Slowly lift both arms forward to chest level, palms facing each other as if embracing a ball, while inhaling deeply (see Illustration 55).

## Focus on Lower Abdomen:

Lightly touch your palms to your chest and abdomen, pressing down slowly while bending the knees into a squat, the focus of the mind also descending with the hands, while exhaling deeply (see Illustration 56).

## Restoration:

Stand naturally upright, letting both arms hang down at the sides of the thighs (refer to Illustration 1).

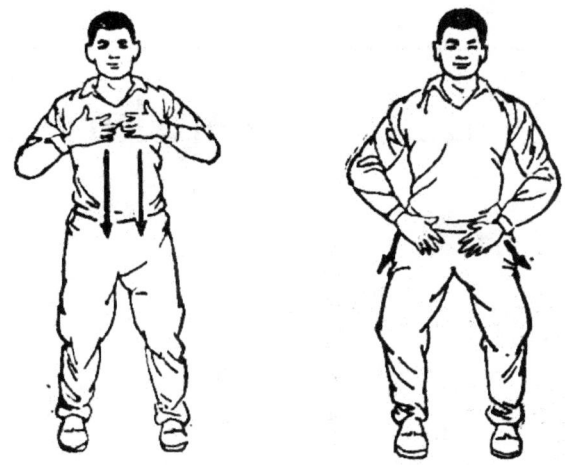

*Illustrations 55 & 56*

# About the Translators

## Master Li Peiyun

Master Li Peiyun, born in China, began his martial arts training at the age of seven. With over five (5) decades of experience in wushu and martial arts, he is one of the few professional Chinese martial artists trained in the classical tradition and in modern methods. He was a member of the prestigious Henan Province Wushu Team and also trained at the Shanghai Physical Education University, the top wushu/physical education university in China. Master Li was not only a top wushu competitor in China but was also trained in the science of wushu and taught to train others in martial arts and healing arts.

## China Competitions

The black and white photo below, taken in 1979, shows Master Li as a member of the prestigious Henan Professional Wushu team. (Master Li is standing third from the right in the back row, next to Chen style tai chi Master Chen Xiaowang (forth from the left).

Many members of this team have become masters in their own right. Notably, the young boy on the far right of the front row is Master Ding Jia, a nine-time consecutive Chen Style Tai Chi Chinese National Champion and Master Li Baoyu (third from the left in the front row). From 1977 through 1990, Master Li actively competed in China, winning numerous gold and silver medals in both weapons and forms.

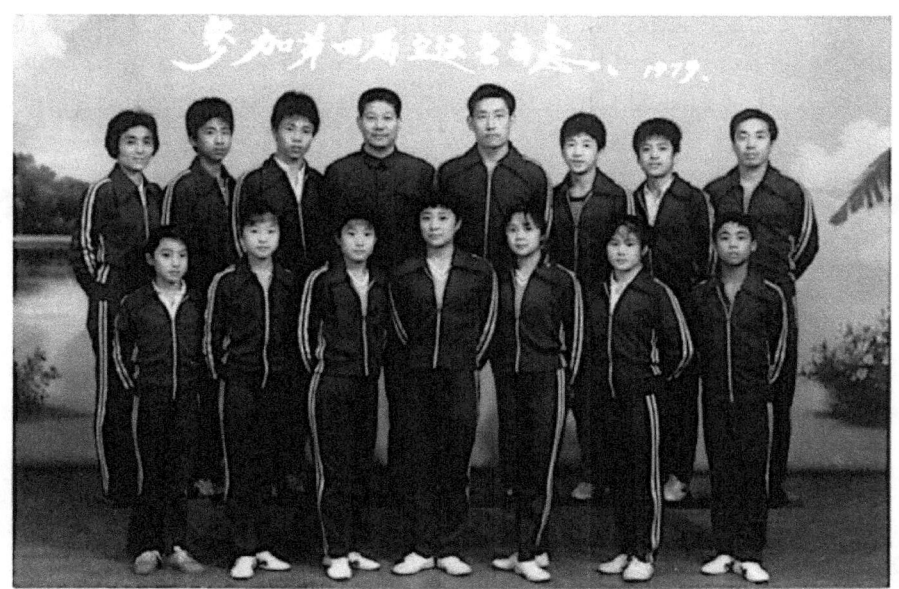

*1979 Henan Professional Wushu Team*

## College Education

Master Li is one of the few professional martial artists to receive formal secondary education in his art. He attended the prestigious Shanghai Physical Education University, graduating first in his class of 400 with a Bachelor of Arts degree in Chinese Martial Arts and Sports Medicine. His university training included advanced instruction in kung-fu theory and styles, basketball, track, soccer, gymnastics, swimming, English, sports pedagogy, theory of sports training, exercise biochemistry, sports biomechanics, anatomy, exercise physiology, weight lifting, sports psychology, sports medicine, traumatology, physical therapy, and massage.

## After College

After earning his degree, Master Li taught at Fudan University in Shanghai from 1993 to 1997. There, he instructed in wushu, tai chi, sports nutrition, soccer, track, basketball, and gymnastics. He also conducted self-defense classes for women and physical therapy classes for disabled students. Master Li coached the Fudan University Kung Fu Team for state competitions and was selected by the Shanghai Kung Fu Association to judge at the highest-ranked Chinese National Kung Fu Tournaments.

## Experience Teaching Young Adults

Master Li has extensive experience training both adults and young adults. He served as the Kung-Fu coach at Shi Hing Chun Elementary School in Shanghai from 1991 to 1993, coaching beginning and intermediate kung fu classes. From 1983 to 1989, he was an instructor of physical education and kung-fu at the Commune for Physical Education in Zhong Yuan City, China, where he selected and coached athletes for state and national kung fu tournaments, taught general physical education classes, and coached the commune's soccer team.

## Relocation to the United States

In April 1997, Master Li relocated to the United States from China and has since become a U.S. citizen. Since Master Li has been in the United States, he has competed nationally and internationally winning grand champion and world titles from organizations such as North American Sport Karate Association (NASKA), National Blackbelt League (NBL), World Kickboxing Association (WKA), and the International Sport Karate Association (ISKA) which was televised on ESPN.

## Establishment of Master Li's Training Center

Master Li established his training center (Master Li's Chinese Martial Arts & Internal Healing Center) in Sewell, New Jersey. It is the premier martial arts training facility in the Tri-State Area. Led personally by Master Li Pei Yun, the center offers a wide range of Chinese martial arts and internal healing practices for both children and adults. The spacious training hall provides ample room for practice, and the center specializes in various disciplines including Wushu (Kung Fu), Tai Chi Chuan (also known as

Taijiquan), Xing Yi and Qigong. The center offers both group and private lessons, serving Southern New Jersey, Philadelphia, and Delaware.

## The Development of Jin Ba Chi®

**Jin Ba Chi®** is a training method developed by Master Li which combines aspects of wushu, tai chi, qigong, yoga, and modern sports science. Master Li begins nearly all Tai Chi classes with a Jin Ba Chi routine to warm up your joints, expand flexibility, increase strength, and improve balance. Master Li has found that combining the Jin Ba Chi conditioning routine with Tai Chi practice helps individuals progress much more quickly than if they simply practice Tai Chi forms alone.

# Kevin Else

Kevin Else's journey in martial arts began with Aikido, which he practiced until lower back injuries necessitated a change. In 1994, he transitioned to Tai Chi Chuan, initially studying under Coach Christopher Pei and Coach Zhang Guifeng at the US Wushu Academy. Since 1998, after moving back to the Philadelphia area, Kevin has been training with Master Li Peiyun at his school (Li's Chinese Martial Arts & Internal Healing Center) in Sewell, New Jersey.

Kevin's expertise spans multiple styles of Tai Chi Chuan and Chinese martial arts, including Yang, Chen, and Sun style Tai Chi, as well as Xing Yi. His dedication to the art has led him to compete internationally, participating in tournaments across the United States, Hong Kong, and mainland China. In 2010, Kevin's skills were recognized when he was named the national Male Internal Martial Arts Competitor of the Year at the U.S. International Kuoshu Championship in Huntsville, Maryland.

Now retired, Kevin dedicates his time to teaching Tai Chi. His unique background allows him to approach the art from both traditional and scientific perspectives. Kevin's mechanical engineering background enables him to analyze Tai Chi postures through the lens of physics and engineering, complementing the deep, traditional knowledge he gained from Master Li. This combination provides him with a comprehensive understanding of Tai Chi and enhances his ability to convey complex concepts to his students.

Kevin's passion for Tai Chi extends beyond practice and teaching. Recognizing the importance of a widely-used Chinese text on Tai Chi Chuan which had never before been translated into English, he was inspired to undertake its translation with Master Li. This project aims to make valuable insights and teachings accessible to a broader, English-speaking audience, further contributing to the global understanding and appreciation of Tai Chi Chuan.

www.ingramcontent.com/pod-product-compliance
Lightning Source LLC
Chambersburg PA
CBHW060459030426
42337CB00015B/1655